MW00387461

CREATING CURIOUS
Young Minds

Jeanne Barker
Kathryn Harvey
Maureen O'Neil
Judy Stewart

revised printing

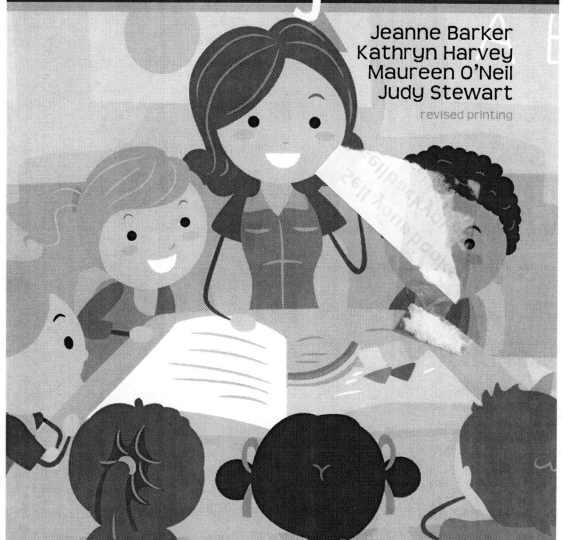

Kendall Hunt
publishing company

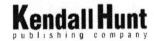

www.kendallhunt.com
Send all inquiries to:
4050 Westmark Drive
Dubuque, IA 52004-1840

Copyright © 2011 by Kendall Hunt Publishing Company

ISBN 978 -1-4652-6875-4

Printed in the United States of America

CONTENTS

Section 3: Physical Development, Health, and Social Science

Section 4: Fine Arts

Supplementary Materials:

ABOUT THE AUTHORS

Jeanne Barker, a retired Associate Professor in Early Childhood Education, was born and raised in Ohio, graduated from Ohio University with both a Bachelor's and Master's Degree in Education. She served as an accrediting member of the Florida Kindergarten Council Board for over 18 years and on the Southern Association of Colleges and Schools Accreditation Committee. Jeanne currently serves on the State of Florida Professional Development Committee. She has taught preschool, been a preschool director, an elementary principal, and now a SCF Professor in early childhood education.

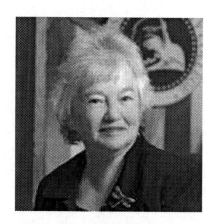

Kathryn Harvey, Assistant Professor in Early Childhood Education at Tallahassee Community College, is a south Florida native. She graduated from Florida State University with a Bachelor's Degree in Visual Arts and a Master's Degree in Early Childhood Education. She is a certified teacher in Florida and previously taught at the pre-K, elementary, middle, and high school levels over a 22-year period. Mrs. Harvey has served on various educational committees, has presented at educational programs and workshops, and has been a teacher mentor. She believes that every child has strengths that are to be nurtured and supported through creative, interactive learning experiences.

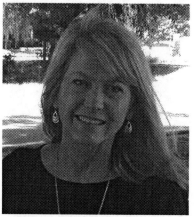

Dr. Maureen O'Neil, Associate Professor, Early Childhood Education, is originally from Connecticut. She has a Doctorate from the School of Education at Boston University. She teaches and directs the early childhood education at Tallahassee Community College. As the Assistant Director of a large non-profit agency, she had the opportunity to supervise the design, curriculum development and certification of a new child care center for children who have witnessed violence. Dr. O'Neil participates in a Service Learning opportunity each semester with early childhood education students at the HOPE Community, a transitional housing program for homeless families. Dr. O'Neil and the students develop lesson plans to use with the children in shelter. She enjoys creating curious young minds through innovative lessons.

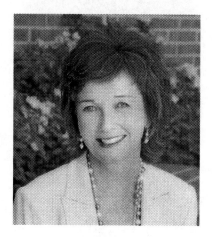

Judy Stewart was born in Wisconsin but completed her high school and college education in Florida. She is an Adjunct Instructor in Early Childhood Education at Tallahassee Community College. A graduate of the University of South Florida, she has a Bachelor's Degree in Elementary and Special Education as well as a Master's Degree in Curriculum and Instruction from the University of Phoenix. Mrs. Stewart is a certified teacher in Florida where she 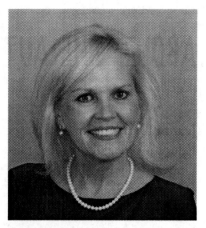 previously taught pre-K, elementary, special education, and high school. She has presented at many teacher workshops and enjoys teaching children how to sing and participate in musical activities.

PREFACE

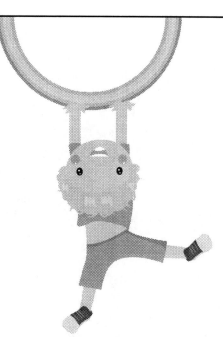

This book is intended for you, the teacher, both new and experienced, to use as a resource manual when planning your lessons, curriculum, or if you are working on local or state early childhood committees. It is designed to be practical, innovative and encourage exploration and creativity in young children. We have also attempted to make it as "user friendly" as possible with a format that is easy to follow.

No resource manual or book can be designed, developed, or completed without the help of some very special people. At Kendall-Hunt Publishing Company, our initial contact was with William England and Doug Kovell. They inspired us to consider writing our resource manual. Karen Snider believed in us from the beginning and encouraged us to do something creative for early childhood teachers and directors. Ashley Schneider has provided feedback, resources, and positive encouragement as the resource manual was being completed. The project has truly been a "team" approach, which has made the process a pleasure to complete.

No book would be complete without saying a special thank you to our families who gave up "family" time for resource manual completion time. Your ability to help us brainstorm creative ideas, understand the scope of the project, and help in any way we asked is sincerely appreciated.

INTRODUCTION

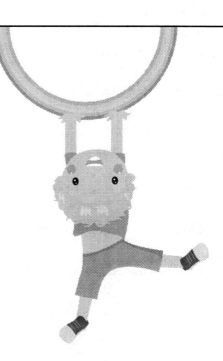

Writing a lesson plan book for educators may not seem important in this day of Internet availability and digital media. However, with the renewed emphasis on the quality of education, teachers and care givers in the field of early childhood are being required to not only update their credentials, but to adopt a set curriculum, and create lesson plans using a set of state adopted standards, goals, and objectives. The formats found on the Internet are many and varied.

Before a teacher or caregiver can even begin to write a lesson plan, there are certain variables that should be considered. These include:

1. Developmentally Appropriate Levels and Practices (DAP)
2. Effective strategies used to teach the lesson plan and how they are developed
3. Whether the content is appropriate
4. Whether the content matches the state standard given for the subject area
5. Whether the lesson plan provides opportunities for diverse learners
   a. Knowledge of the diverse learners
   b. Adjustments needed and how they will be designed and implemented.

Once the variables have been defined, it is then up to the teacher to be able to apply the lesson in the group setting.

A lesson plan is just one of the many teaching tools used in early childhood education but one that has suddenly taken on academic importance in this field. With the passage of early childhood voluntary prekindergarten mandates in many states, suddenly attention was focused on quality of child care education, not just day care. State child care requirements were upgraded for child care professionals as well as their directors. Community colleges, four-year colleges and universities, changed their courses to reflect curriculum evaluation and lesson plan training, as well as including lesson plans as part of their field experience.

There are many educational resources available that include lesson plan development from the NAEYC sample lesson plan to many types of lesson plans available through the Internet and publishing companies nationwide. It is important to create a lesson plan outline that meets the needs of your program, the state requirements, and the developmental level of the children.

An example would be:

Title of Lesson – Title should reflect the subject of the lesson plan and should be innovative and creative.

Goal – Overall goal of what you want to accomplish in the lesson plan.

Objective – Specific objective of the lesson plan should be stated.

Developmental Domain – Of the following list, which of the domains will be met?
       Physical
       Social/Emotional
       Language and Communication
       Cognitive
       Creative

Materials Needed – What do you need to teach and apply the lesson?

Environment – Where will the lesson be presented and to what size group?

Procedure – Step by step procedure of presenting the lesson plan with follow-through.

Questions for the Children – Appropriate questions for children that correspond with the lesson. (These can be included with the procedure.)

Lesson Extension Ideas – How could you enrich the lesson beyond the initial scope of the plan?

How to Check for Student Understanding – What method will you use to determine the level of understanding gained for each child?

Accommodations for Diverse Learners – What activities, procedures, or adjustments will you make to meet the needs of diverse learners?

Evaluation of the Lesson – What criteria will you use to evaluate the lesson?

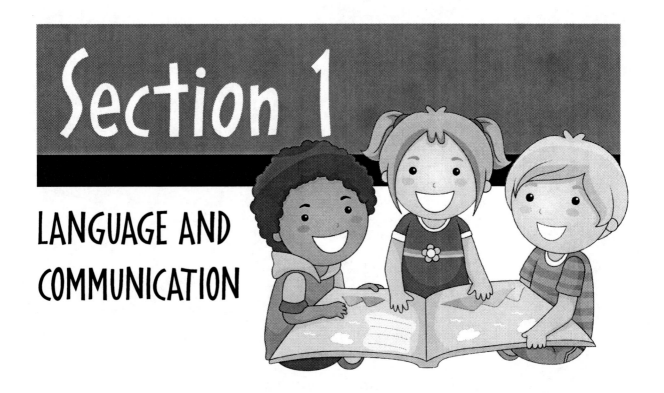

Section 1

LANGUAGE AND COMMUNICATION

The development of language and communication skills is an integral part of a young child's development. As children develop, language emerges; this emergent process is greatly enhanced when children are exposed to a language-rich environment. Statistics show that the earlier and the more we expose children to language and literature, the better they are able to develop in all areas. It is important to understand that through language children are able to build cognitive associations that help them understand the meaning of information. Language acquisition also significantly affects social and emotional development as children make connections with others while expressing their needs and interests. They gain knowledge that can help them understand themselves, others, and the world around them.

The lessons and activities in this section have been used successfully to move children forward in their development through stories, discussion, process, and reflection. They have been designed to encourage children to ask questions, express themselves, create new outcomes, and interact cooperatively with others. Adjustments can be made to simplify or challenge depending on the age and developmental levels of the children you are teaching. The confidence that children can gain as they learn how to understand and use language is a lifelong benefit we want every child to enjoy!

ACTIVITY 1

BEAR CAVES

> ### GOAL:
> To expose children to the concept of hibernation.
>
> ### OBJECTIVE:
> The children will dictate bear facts and create a three-dimensional bear and cave habitat.

Developmental Domain(s) Met:

Physical – Fine motor; molding clay, drawing, and gluing.
Language and Communication – Child dictates to describe their bear habitat.
Creative – Interpreting their idea using various materials.

Materials Needed:

* A book about bears and hibernation
* Photos of bears in their natural habitat
* Children's scissors
* Markers or crayons
* Craft glue
* Five or six cotton balls per child (for snow)
* One small piece of modeling clay per child (for bears)
* One small Styrofoam bowl per child (for caves)
* One 9 x 12 sheet of heavy construction paper or cardboard per child

Environment (Indoor/Outdoor, Size of Group):

Indoor, group size 8 to 12 (this activity is best with 4-year-olds and older).

Procedure and Questions: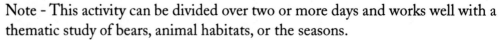

Note - This activity can be divided over two or more days and works well with a thematic study of bears, animal habitats, or the seasons.

- Read the story to the children.
- Ask open-ended questions that help the children discuss facts about bears and their habits. Include questions about what bears eat and when, and why the bears go into a cave.
- Explain that each child is going to make their own bear and bear cave habitat.

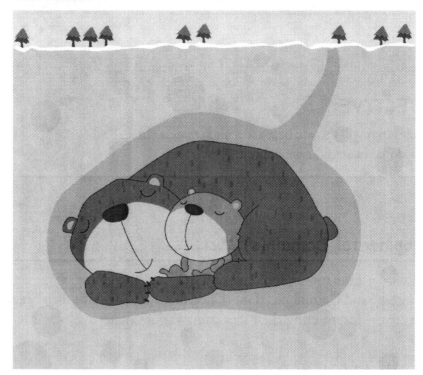

Model the project in front of the children.

1. Fold the 9 x 12 paper in half and make a crease.
2. On one side of the crease color green grass, berries, flowers and/or a blue stream with fish to represent spring.
3. Take the Styrofoam bowl, turn it upside down and cut two "cave entrances" opposite each other from the bowl.
4. Glue the "cave" down on the paper with one entrance facing the spring side of the paper and the other facing the winter side of the paper.
5. Show the children how to spread out cotton balls and glue them down on the side of the crease opposite spring to represent winter.
6. Mold a simple bear out of a small piece of modeling clay and show the children that the bear will eat their fill, go into the cave, sleep through the cold winter, and come out hungry in the spring.

7. Let each child look at the model, and then put it away so that they will create their own interpretation.
8. While children are working on their habitat, let each one dictate a fact or story about their bear to you. They can either write it later themselves or you can type it for them. When the project is complete, glue or attach their words to the habitat.

LESSON EXTENSION IDEAS:
- In a corner of your room create a bear cave with sheets.
- Have a pajamas-and-teddy-bears day allowing the children to bring a teddy bear (or favorite stuffed animal) to school for the day. Sort the bears by size, color, and type. Sing the "teddy bear" song!
- Provide bear sorting and counting manipulatives.
- Provide books and puzzles about bears.

HOW TO CHECK FOR STUDENT UNDERSTANDING: Understanding can be checked by responses to open-ended questions and by the fact or story dictation they provide.

ACCOMMODATIONS FOR DIVERSE LEARNERS (SPECIAL NEEDS):
Provide one-on-one guidance; simplify the process with just a cave and a bear; provide bear figures and a teacher-prepared winter/spring play mat.

EVALUATION OF THE LESSON: You will observe the different ability levels of the children and determine time needed for the multi-step process to be completed. If a child becomes frustrated, allow others to help or reduce the number of steps involved (see "Accommodations for diverse learners" above).

ACTIVITY 2

COOPERATIVE BOOK REPORTS

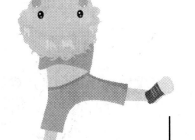

GOAL:
To expose children to the excitement of books.

OBJECTIVE:
With a partner, the children will choose a book to read or listen to and explain to others.

Developmental Domain(s) Met:

Physical – Fine motor: holding a book correctly and turning the pages.
Social/Emotional – Working with a partner cooperatively.
Language and Communication – Explaining the book they chose to others.
Cognitive – Left to right, top to bottom progression.

Materials Needed:

* A collection of developmentally appropriate children's picture books.

Environment (Indoor/Outdoor, Size of Group):

Indoor, group size 8 to 12 (this activity is best with 4-year-olds and older).

Procedure and Questions:

- You will model the correct way to read a book to the children with an adult assistant. Take turns talking, pointing, and turning pages.
- Use voice inflection, character voices, and pauses while you read.
- Each of you should take a turn telling the children what you liked about the book.
- Ask the children if they have any questions about the book.

- Explain to the children that with a partner they will choose a book they both like, read it or have it read to them, and then read and/or explain it to the class.
- Remind them that they both have to like the book.
- Give the children time to choose a book. As time allows throughout the day or week have each pair come up to share their book.

LESSON EXTENSION IDEAS:
- Offer the children props and/or puppets to use while telling their story.
- Have the children draw their favorite character or scene in the story to display in the classroom.

HOW TO CHECK FOR STUDENT UNDERSTANDING: Record the reading, explanation, and listening skills of each child.

ACCOMMODATIONS FOR DIVERSE LEARNERS (SPECIAL NEEDS): None.

EVALUATION OF THE LESSON: The teacher will evaluate the activity by observing the children's enjoyment of both telling the story and listening to the stories.

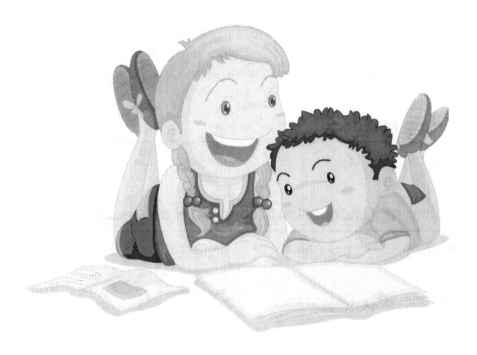

ACTIVITY 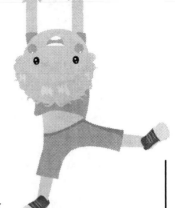 3

CREATIVE & COOPERATIVE WRITING

GOAL:

To create an awareness of story structure.

OBJECTIVE:

The children will contribute to a cooperative story through dictation and illustrations.

Developmental Domain(s) Met:

Physical – Fine motor; drawing with oil pastels.
Social/Emotional – Cooperative story creation.
Language and Communication – Verbalizing story concepts.
Cognitive – Story sequencing and development.
Creative – Interpreting and drawing their idea artistically. Using their imagination in story creation.

Materials Needed:

* A children's Caldecott Award winning picture book
* Large chart paper
* Easel
* Notepad
* Markers
* Construction paper in a variety of colors
* Oil pastels (Oil pastels on colored construction paper create a vibrant picture!)

Environment (Indoor/Outdoor, Size of Group):

Indoor, group size 8 to 12 (this activity is best with 4-year-olds and older).

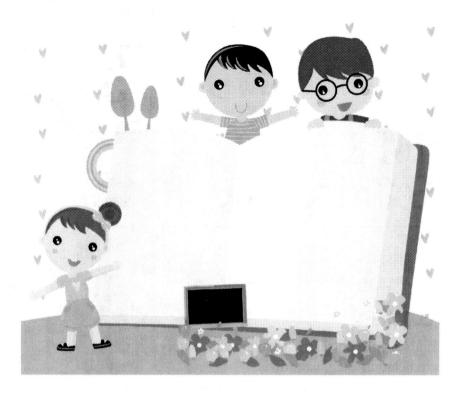

Procedure:

- Show the children the Caldecott storybook. Point out that this particular story was chosen to win an award because the pictures and story work so well together.
- Read the book to the children. Explain that storybooks have a plot (what the story is about) and that each story has at least one person, place, or thing (characters and places) in the plot, using those in the story as the example.
- Have each child choose one person, place, or thing; write down what they chose on your notepad with their name. Note: It's best to steer them away from using a character they're already familiar with such as the Little Mermaid or SpongeBob because they will already have a preconceived notion of that character.
- Ask them how they would like to begin their story and write what they say on the large chart paper with colorful markers to keep their attention. Then one by one ask each child what their person, place, or thing is doing in the story. You may have to guide them some by asking them questions as you write their story.
- Once you have included all characters or places, help them wrap up the story with a conclusion.

Questions for Children:

To help them use descriptive words –
- What is your character doing?
- What does it look like?
- Why do you want a . . . [lake, mountain, car, spaceship (their idea)] in the story?
- Where is your character from or going?

LESSON EXTENSION IDEAS: Have the children illustrate their person, place, or thing on construction paper with oil pastels. If they are able to, help them write a title for their drawing.

The completed story can be posted on the wall with the illustrations placed around it. The story can also be typed and placed in a class book with the children's illustrations.

This can be done with several classes and the teachers "vote" on the award-winning story, of course they all win at an "awards ceremony" and each story gets a gold sticker!

HOW TO CHECK FOR STUDENT UNDERSTANDING: The teacher will check for understanding by determining if each child was able to contribute an interconnected idea to the story.

ACCOMMODATIONS FOR DIVERSE LEARNERS (SPECIAL NEEDS): Diverse learners and younger children can contribute to the story by working with them one on one to develop the story ideas. Props and listening centers can be used to reinforce the concept of plot, character, and setting.

EVALUATION OF THE LESSON: The teacher will evaluate the lesson by reviewing the completed story and checking to determine if the children could create a cohesive story line.

ACTIVITY 4

I CAN RHYME

GOAL:

To help children understand what makes a word rhyme.

OBJECTIVE:

The children will see objects that rhyme and say rhyming words.

Developmental Domain(s) Met:

Language and Communication – Ending sound recognition.
Cognitive – Learning to differentiate the sounds that rhyme from those that do not rhyme.

Materials Needed:

* A short rhyming book
* Small manipulatives that rhyme with each other
  (e.g., mouse/house, goat/boat, clock/block, hat/cat, bug/rug, frog/dog, bee/tree, fish/dish, spoon/moon)
* Additional random items that do not rhyme
* A tray or flat surface to display rhyming items

Environment (Indoor/Outdoor, Size of Group):

Indoor, group size 8 to 12.

Procedure and Questions:

* Read the rhyming book emphasizing the ending sounds that rhyme.
* Ask the children if they know what words rhymed and why.

- Ask the children if they can say two rhyming words (silly words should be accepted).
- Show the children all of the manipulatives on a tray or table randomly placed. Ask them to help you find two that have rhyming names; continue until all matches are found. Be sure to hold and say the names of non-rhyming items while emphasizing the ending sounds and the difference in sound.
- To recap have the children say each rhyming pair in unison as you hold them up.

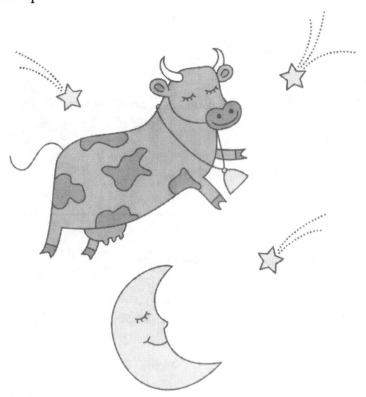

LESSON EXTENSION IDEAS: Set up a center with the rhyming manipulatives for children to play with. Read the nursery rhyme "Hey Diddle Diddle" and let the children play with dishes and spoons.

HOW TO CHECK FOR STUDENT UNDERSTANDING: Work with children one on one to check for ending-sound rhyming. Keep a checklist on each child while you observe them as they say the rhyming words.

ACCOMMODATIONS FOR DIVERSE LEARNERS (SPECIAL NEEDS): Allow children to hold the manipulatives as you say the words. Say just the ending sound in isolation.

EVALUATION OF THE LESSON: The lesson should be fun! You will observe different ability levels. This will help you in your lesson planning as you expose children to words and sounds.

ACTIVITY 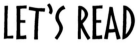 5

LET'S READ

GOAL:
To get parents involved in reading with their child.

OBJECTIVE:
The children along with their parents will complete a "Read-a-thon" of at least six books.

Developmental Domain(s) Met:

Physical – Children will use fine motor skills to manipulate the books and turn the pages.

Social/Emotional – Children will bond with their parents through interaction while reading together.

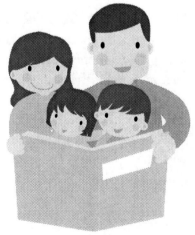

Language and Communication – Children will talk to each other, to the teacher, and to their parents about the book topics.

Cognitive – Children will understand that books can have a beginning, a middle, and an end. Children will help develop questions for a question sheet.

Creative – Children will use dramatic play to tell their favorite story. In the art center children can design their own book bag. Children will use their imaginations to create various endings to the story.

Materials Needed:

* Chart with "Read-a-thon" dates
* Sample selection of books for the children to choose

Environment (Indoor/Outdoor, Size of Group):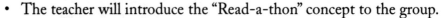

Small group at the beginning of no more than six; begin indoors in the "reading nook" center.

Procedure and Questions:

- The teacher will introduce the "Read-a-thon" concept to the group.
- The teacher will ask the children if they would like to participate in a contest called a "Read-a-thon" and read with their parents (at least six books in six weeks).
- The children will bring a special book bag to transport the book they will take home each week.
- The children will make a list of questions each week to ask the parents about their book (for example, did you like this book? Why or why not? If you were the author of this book, how would you want it to end?).

ACCOMMODATIONS FOR DIVERSE LEARNERS: If possible include books on tape or large print books that are developmentally appropriate for the child.

LESSON EXTENSION IDEAS: Have a Friday night open house where the children could perform a puppet show about their favorite books, dress up as a storybook character, or simply share how it worked in their family setting.

HOW TO CHECK FOR STUDENT UNDERSTANDING: The children will return the book each Monday morning with a question sheet completed about the book they read. The teacher will ask the children if they read with their parent(s) and if they can share the answers to the questions about their book.

EVALUATION OF THE LESSON: Teacher will evaluate the lesson each week based on the number of children who successfully read at least one book with their parent(s) and answered the question sheet.

ACTIVITY 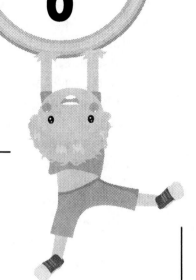 6

MY STORY APRON

GOAL:

To enhance storytelling skills and creativity.

OBJECTIVE:

The children will make their own story apron.

Developmental Domain(s) Met:

Physical – Fine motor: gluing and tying.
Social/Emotional – Oral presentation to others.
Language and Communication – Using books and self expression.
Creative – Creating original stories.

Materials Needed:

* One 9 x 12 and one 9 x 6 piece of colored felt per child
* Children's scissors
* Ribbon
* Craft glue
* Props, cut-outs, and books for storytelling
* Various buttons and scraps

Environment (Indoor/Outdoor, Size of Group):

Indoor, group size 8 to 12 (this activity is best with 4-year-olds and older).

Procedure:

- Tell an Apron Story to your class using props and a book.
- Explain that each child will make their own story apron.

1. Holding a 9 x 12 piece of felt vertically, model how to fold the felt to cut one small slit in each top corner and one small slit on each side of the felt near the edges.

2. Push a piece of ribbon through each slit and demonstrate how to tie a knot making the neck straps and waist straps.

3. Using the half piece of felt, glue along two short edges and one long edge and place on top of the lower half of the 9 x 12 piece that you have attached the ribbon to (make sure it is open on the top, creating a large pocket).

4. Decorate the apron using glue, buttons, and scraps.

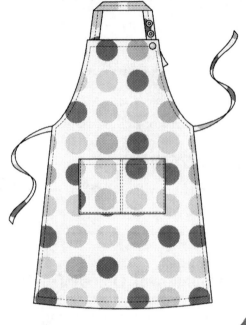

Questions for Children:

- What can you put in your apron pocket?
- What story would you like to tell?
- Would you like to use a book or make up a story?

LESSON EXTENSION IDEAS: Children can use the pockets to hold props, figures, and animals, and create an imaginative story of their own.
Children can play a game with their friends, "What's in my pocket?" and give clues for others to guess what they have in the pocket.

HOW TO CHECK FOR STUDENT UNDERSTANDING: Observe students as they prepare and use the story apron to tell a story of their choosing.

ACCOMMODATIONS FOR DIVERSE LEARNERS (SPECIAL NEEDS): Assist students with cutting and tying as needed. For those with social limitations, work with them in small groups.

EVALUATION OF THE LESSON: The effectiveness of the lesson will be judged on the utilization of the aprons, the imaginative play, and the interaction with others.

ACTIVITY 7

OUR CLASS LIBRARY

GOAL:

To expose children to early reader books.

OBJECTIVE:

The children will be introduced to the process of reading and checking out classroom books that will continue throughout the school year.

Developmental Domain(s) Met:

Physical – Fine motor; handling books.
Social/Emotional – Paired reading with adults and other children.
Language and Communication – Oral reading and story discussion.
Cognitive – Ability to follow a sequence of directions.

Materials Needed:

* Early Predictable Reader Books (label each book with a number on the outside)
* A master list of each book with the corresponding number
* A checkout list or spreadsheet to write the book number next to the name of the child. This helps to keep track of which and how many books each child has read.
* Plastic protective baggies for books (zip-lock bags work well)
* A mobile book basket (this is helpful so that books can be checked out during free play and outside times)
* A label on the back of each book to explain to the parent what the child's responsibility is. E.g., "Your child has brought home this book to encourage, enhance, and build confidence in their reading skills. Please have them read this Predictable Reader book to you, to their stuffed animals, siblings, grandparents, and/or friends. Your excitement will

promote their progress! Please remind them to place it back in the bag provided and return to school to check out another book."

Environment (Indoor/Outdoor, Size of Group):

Indoor, group size 8 to 12 for introduction of books. One-on-one for book check-out (this activity is best with 4-year-olds and older).

Procedure:

- Show the predictable readers to the children. Read one to them, and let them read to you. Express excitement at their ability to "read," how wonderful reading is and why! Repeat with a second book.
- Ask the children how they would take care of a book. Let them know that it is not good to leave the books around pets, babies, food, or water!
- Explain to children that:
    - Each child will check out a book to read at home after first reading one to you.
    - Once they finish reading to any and everyone at home, they are to put the book back in the baggie and place it where they will remember it when they leave for school.
    - They are to drop the book in the book return box in your classroom; once the books have been checked in, they will be able to check out another!

While the children are at centers call one child at a time, let them choose a book, read it to them, then have them "read" it back to you. Give positive feedback for all reading levels. Log in the book number and let them take the book home!

Questions for Children:

- During one-on-one time ask the children if they remember what they are to do with the book.
- How they will take care of it?
- Who is responsible for returning it, and where they will return it to?

LESSON EXTENSION IDEAS:
- Children can have a show-n-tell book time and explain their favorite book to the class.
- Have a reading reward treasure box for each five books read.

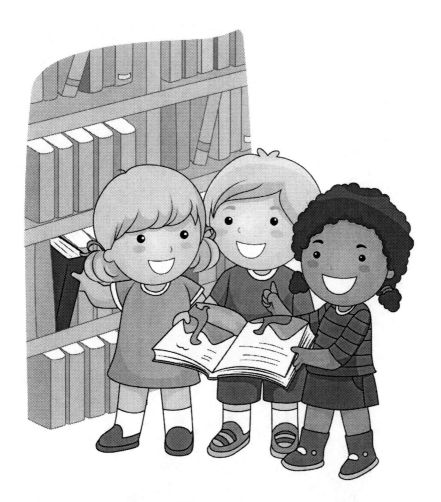

HOW TO CHECK FOR STUDENT UNDERSTANDING: Keeping a record of who checks out books and how many are checked out throughout the year will provide information on ability to follow directions as well as on reading development.

ACCOMMODATIONS FOR DIVERSE LEARNERS (SPECIAL NEEDS): Create a visual cue card to remind children of what to do with the books. Introduce wordless picture books to children as well as books with words. Have the children read to a volunteer, an aide, or another teacher if they have any challenges regarding taking books home to read.

EVALUATION OF THE LESSON: Although preparation of the class library takes a little while, it can be used repeatedly throughout the year and is a wonderful confidence builder for young readers.

Once the initial introduction of the class library is done, it is easy to have an aide or class volunteer check books out to the children. Over time you can evaluate the usage and interest. In a preschool program of 60 children, you will want to have 40 – 60 predictable reader books in your library (these can be bought in sets and will last for years).

ACTIVITY **8**

THE VERY BEAUTIFUL BUTTERFLY

(a story extension of "The Very Hungry Caterpillar"
by Eric Carle)

GOAL:

To expose children to the concept of metamorphosis.

OBJECTIVE:

The children will listen and retell the story, act out
the story and extend the story.

Developmental Domain(s) Met:

> Physical – Fine motor: painting. Gross motor: movement (acting out
> the story).
> Cognitive – Story sequencing.
> Language and Communication – Dictation of the story.
> Creative – Story development.

Materials Needed:

* Book - *The Very Hungry Caterpillar*, by Eric Carle
* Paint
* Art paper

Environment (Indoor/Outdoor, Size of Group):

Indoor and outdoor, group size 8 to 12 (this activity is best with 4-year-olds
and older).

Procedure and Questions:

* Read the story, pausing and letting the children respond throughout.
* Ask the children to retell the story in order of events.

- Introduce and emphasize words: chrysalis, cocoon, and metamorphosis.
- Take the children outside and have them pretend they are the caterpillar acting out spinning a cocoon, transforming, and coming out of the cocoon as a butterfly.
- Have the children paint their own "Very Beautiful Butterfly."
- Ask the children to tell you what they think happened to the beautiful butterfly after it came out of the cocoon.
- Write their words on a sentence strip or paper to put with their art.

LESSON EXTENSION IDEAS:
- Set up props to retell the story.
- Create a book out of the student's words and art.
- Go on a nature walk and look for a chrysalis or cocoon.
- Keep a butterfly habitat in your classroom to observe the metamorphosis.
- Grow a butterfly garden.

HOW TO CHECK FOR STUDENT UNDERSTANDING: Ask the children to retell the story. Observe gross motor control while acting out metamorphosis and fine motor control in painting. Document their ability to develop the story creatively.

ACCOMMODATIONS FOR DIVERSE LEARNERS (SPECIAL NEEDS): Break the lesson into smaller segments over a longer period of time. Have props for hands on experience.

EVALUATION OF THE LESSON: The teacher will evaluate the activity based on student participation, responses to story reflection, creativity, and enjoyment.

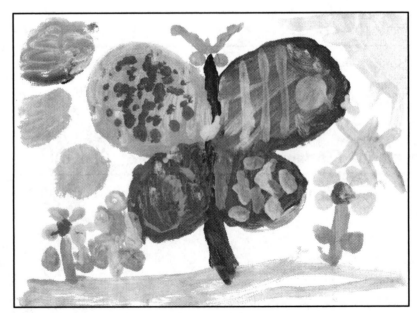

ACTIVITY 9

WE CAN WRITE A SONG

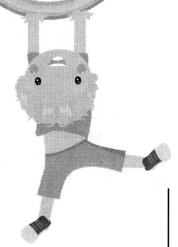

GOAL:

To expose children to the concept of putting their own words to music.

OBJECTIVE:

The children will add words to a familiar tune to create their own song.

Developmental Domain(s) Met:

Social/Emotional – Cooperative song development.

Language and Communication – Contributing words and ideas for the song.

Creative – Using their imagination to develop cohesive lyrics.

Materials Needed:

* CD player and a CD of children's songs
* Easel paper
* Markers
* Read a book based on a theme that you are studying (Grandparent's Day, Valentine's Day, Shapes, Dinosaurs. . .)

Environment (Indoor/Outdoor, Size of Group):

Indoor, group size 8 to 12 (this activity is best with 4-year-olds and older).

Procedure and Questions:

- Read the book you have chosen that matches your theme.
- Ask the children open-ended questions about the book.
- Play familiar songs on the CD player.
- Ask the children what words they heard in the songs.
- Tell the children that they will be writing their own song about . . . [your theme].
- Write down what the children tell you (silly songs can be fun too). For example:

> My grandpa wears glasses and reads to me.
> I call my grandma Gigi.
> My Gigi takes me to the store.
> My grandpa buys me ice cream.
> He helps me ride my bicycle.
> We love our grandparents and they love us.

(This can be sung to Twinkle, Twinkle Little Star or Mary Had a Little Lamb.)

- Once you have written all of their words, you will have one or more verses.
- Sing the song to the children and help them learn it. It won't take long, it's their words!

LESSON EXTENSION IDEAS:
- Set up an art center where children can illustrate the lyrics to the song.
- Set up a time when the children can sing for others.
- Send a written copy home with each child.
- Use other song tunes.

HOW TO CHECK FOR STUDENT UNDERSTANDING: If they contribute words and ideas and they sing along – they understand!

ACCOMMODATIONS FOR DIVERSE LEARNERS (SPECIAL NEEDS):
For children with hearing impairment, use rhythmic instruments for them to feel the beat.

EVALUATION OF THE LESSON: Determine if the children were able to contribute to the lyrics while staying within the boundary of the theme and if they enjoyed the process as well as singing their song!

ACTIVITY 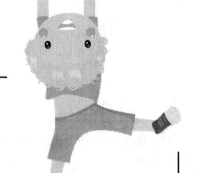 10

WHAT'S MISSING?

GOAL:

To use memorization and communication skills.

OBJECTIVE:

The children will be able to identify objects and recall the objects after they are removed.

Developmental Domain(s) Met:

Social/Emotional – The children will learn to take turns while others are speaking.

Language and Communication – The children will be able to label objects and tell what they are used for.

Cognitive – The children will be able to count objects and identify what they are.

Materials Needed:

 A large tray

 6-8 small objects (e.g., healthy/unhealthy snacks, farm animals, holiday toys, cars/trucks, items that start with the letter A,B,C)

Environment (Indoor/Outdoor, Size of Group):

Small group in the classroom seated on the floor. Make sure each child can see the tray of items clearly.

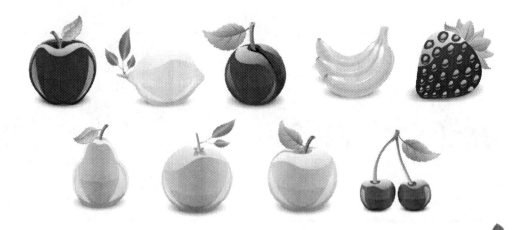

Procedure:

The teacher will begin the lesson by showing the children the items on the tray. She will ask them to identify each one and tell what it is used for. The class will count the number of items together. The children will close their eyes as the teacher removes an item and hides it behind back. When the teacher says, "open," the children open their eyes and tell what has been removed. The teacher repeats this procedure until all items are removed. (May remove more than one item at a time.)

Questions for Children:

- What are these items?
- What are they used for?
- How many items are on the tray?
- Which one is your favorite?
- What item was removed from the tray?

LESSON EXTENSION IDEAS: The lesson could be extended by having the children get into groups of two or three and play this game with each other.

HOW TO CHECK FOR STUDENT UNDERSTANDING: The teacher will evaluate the students by checking counting skills, identification skills, verbal skills, and memorization skills.

ACCOMMODATIONS FOR DIVERSE LEARNERS (SPECIAL NEEDS): Students with special needs should sit close to the teacher and be given additional time to recall missing items.

EVALUATION OF THE LESSON: The teacher will evaluate the lesson based on student enjoyment and participation in the activity.

Section 2

MATH AND SCIENCE

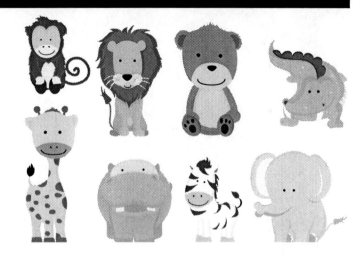

Math and Science have become increasingly important subjects in the preschool curriculum. Children who do not have a basic understanding of math and science concepts will find it much more difficult to keep up with the rigorous pace in a kindergarten curriculum. Math and Science readiness activities are becoming more and more common in preschools and childcare centers.

The Math and Science activities found in this resource manual are designed to give teachers hands-on and ready-to-use activities. Many of the concepts may seem very simple but children need to master these basic building blocks before they can successfully move on to more complex ideas. Each lesson is designed to not only present a particular topic but also to encourage the children to use their imaginations and creativity. Each lesson is also designed to be fun as well as educational and should encourage exploration and discovery.

ACTIVITY 1

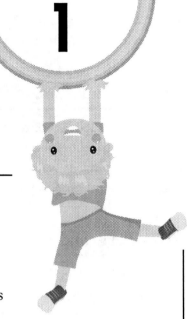

AM I A BIRD?

GOAL:

To understand life science.

OBJECTIVE:

The children will be able to identify that all birds have feathers.

Note: For the purpose of this lesson, as long as it has feathers, it's a bird.

Developmental Domain(s) Met:
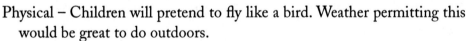

Physical – Children will pretend to fly like a bird. Weather permitting this would be great to do outdoors.

Social/Emotional – The children will be put in groups of two and will look at various animals that can fly and decide if they are a bird. Various animals such as a bat, a butterfly, and a ladybug should be used to distinguish that just because you can fly, doesn't mean you are a bird.

Language and Communication – Children will talk to their partner and to the teacher about why an animal is or is not a bird.

Cognitive – Children will be exposed to various animals that can fly. The children must determine whether or not the animal is a bird by whether or not it has feathers.

Creative – After the children view the various types of animals that can fly, they will be asked to draw their own bird. For the purpose of this lesson, as long as their drawing has feathers, it's a bird.

Materials Needed:

* Book – *Birds of a Feather* by Vanita Oelschlager and Robin Hegan
* Pictures of various animals such as a bat, ladybug, and a butterfly (Bird Supplement #1)

* Examples of feathers (available at craft stores)
* Paper and crayons

Note: If you have a local bird association, you can try to arrange for them to come to your class for this lesson.

Environment (Indoor/Outdoor, Size of Group):

Indoor or outdoor is appropriate. If weather permits, teachers may want to take children outside to look at birds in their area. Children will explore in groups of two (or three if necessary) and number of teachers depends on your state teacher/student ratio requirements.

Procedure and Questions:

Teacher will explain that all birds have feathers but not all things that can fly are birds. For this lesson, we will not focus on other aspects of bird anatomy.

* Teacher will read the book, *Birds of a Feather* and emphasize the feathers whenever possible.
* Then the teacher will pass around sample feathers so the children can see and feel them.
* Teachers will ask children if they are birds and how do they know.
* Show the children pictures of other animals that can fly and ask the children to explain why they are not birds even though they can fly.

The children will have the opportunity to be creative and draw their own bird. For this lesson, as long as the drawing has feathers, it is a bird.

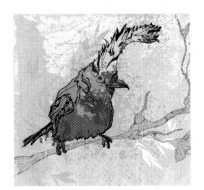

ACCOMMODATIONS FOR DIVERSE LEARNERS (SPECIAL NEEDS): All children should be included in this activity regardless of special needs.

LESSON EXTENSION IDEAS: Books on the topic of birds should be available in the classroom reading center. In the manipulative center, have feathers available for the children to examine. Art center activities should include pictures of various birds.

HOW TO CHECK FOR STUDENT UNDERSTANDING: The teacher will have pictures of various animals that can fly and will ask the students if they are birds. The children should know that the animals with feathers are birds.

EVALUATION OF THE LESSON: Teachers can evaluate the lesson based on the number of children who could identify whether or not an animal was a bird based on whether or not it had feathers.

ACTIVITY 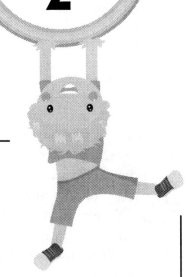 2

AM I A BUG?

> ### GOAL:
>
> To understand life science.
>
> ### OBJECTIVE:
>
> The children will be able to identify that all bugs must have six legs.

Developmental Domain(s) Met:

Physical – Children will go on a nature walk and see if they can find a bug.

Social/Emotional – The children will be put in groups of two to look for bugs and discuss why what they find is or is not a bug.

Language and Communication – Children will talk to their partner and to the teacher about why something is or is not a bug.

Cognitive – Children must be able to count to six to decide if something is or is not a bug.

Creative – After the children explore, have them draw their own kind of bug. For the purpose of this lesson, as long as it has six legs, it is a bug.

Materials Needed:

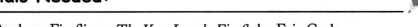

* Book on Fireflies – *The Very Lonely Firefly* by Eric Carle
* Some type of pointer (such as straws) so children can point to objects they find without risking being stung or bit by a bug or insect
* Paper and crayons
* Magnifying glasses

Environment (Indoor/Outdoor, Size of Group):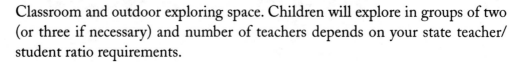

Classroom and outdoor exploring space. Children will explore in groups of two (or three if necessary) and number of teachers depends on your state teacher/student ratio requirements.

Procedure:

Teacher will explain that all bugs have six legs. For this lesson, we will not focus on other aspects of bug anatomy.

- Teacher will read the book on fireflies and emphasize the six legs whenever possible.
- Ask children whether or not they are bugs and how do they know.
- Children and teacher(s) will then go outside and point to various objects and ask if it is a bug. If it has six legs, it is a bug. This activity is best done at a time when bugs are present outside.
- Children can examine things with the magnifying glasses to determine if they are bugs.
- Teachers should emphasize that children should not actually touch the things they find with their hands, just the pointer or straw.
- Teachers will also emphasize respecting nature and they should not hurt or squish any living thing.
- When children come back to the classroom, they will discuss what they saw and whether or not they found any bugs.
- Give students the opportunity to be creative and draw their own bug. For this lesson, as long as the drawing has six legs, it is a bug.

Questions for Children:

When the teacher reads the book, ask the children how many legs a bug has several times to reinforce it.

The teacher may ask:
- A spider has eight legs, is it a bug?
- A dog has four legs, is it a bug?
- A person has two legs, is it a bug?
- A bird has two legs and wings, is it a bug?
- A snake has no legs, is it a bug?

The teacher can ask as many of these questions as desired.

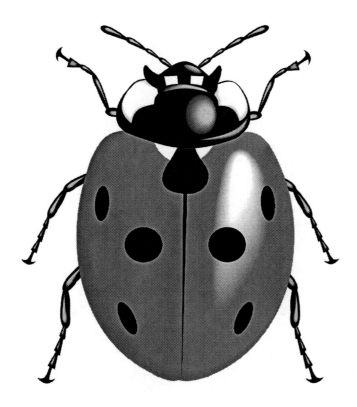

ACCOMMODATIONS FOR DIVERSE LEARNERS (SPECIAL NEEDS):
All children should be included in this activity regardless of special needs. If you have students with mobility issues, they should be able to navigate the outdoor space. For a gifted student, have pictures of animals with more than six legs, such as a spider, an octopus, or a centipede and the children can count the legs.

LESSON EXTENSION IDEAS: Books on the topic of insects should be available in the reading center. In the manipulative center, the focus should be on counting to the number six. Art center activities should include pictures of various insects. In the kitchen center, children can be exposed to common foods that come from insects, such as honey.

HOW TO CHECK FOR STUDENT UNDERSTANDING: The teacher will have a picture of an animal with no legs (snake), a two-legged, and a four legged animal and ask the children if they are bugs. The children should be able to distinguish that if it has six legs, it is a bug and if does not have six legs, it is not a bug.

EVALUATION OF THE LESSON: Teachers can evaluate the lesson based on the number of children who could identify whether or not an animal was a bug based on the number of legs.

ACTIVITY 3

AM I A FISH?

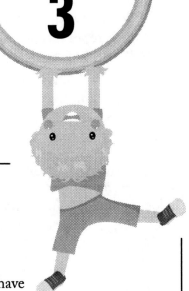

GOAL:

To understand life science.

OBJECTIVE:

The children will be able to identify that all fish have fins and that things other than fish can swim.

Note: For the purpose of this lesson, as long as it has fins, it's a fish.

Developmental Domain(s) Met:

Physical – Children will pretend to swim like a human and then pretend to swim like a fish. When swimming like a human, the children should lay on the floor and the teacher will demonstrate how to do the freestyle stroke. When pretending to swim like a fish, they will again lay on the floor while holding their arms close to their bodies and just use their hands like fins.

Social/Emotional – The children will be put in groups of two and will look at various animals and decide if they are a fish.

Language and Communication – Children will talk to their partner and to the teacher about why an animal is or is not a fish.

Cognitive – Children will be exposed to various animals that can swim. The children must determine whether or not the animal is using fins to swim and therefore, is or is not a fish.

Creative – After the children view the various types of animals that can swim, they will be asked to draw their own fish. For the purpose of this lesson, as long as their drawing has fins, it's a fish.

Materials Needed:

* Book on Fish – *The Rainbow Fish* by Marcus Pfister
* Pictures of various fish
* Pictures of other animals that can swim such as a duck, a turtle, and a human (Supplement #1)
* Paper and crayons

Note: It is beneficial if the classroom has an aquarium but it is not required.

Environment (Indoor/Outdoor, Size of Group):

Indoor or outdoor is appropriate. Children will explore in groups of two (or three if necessary) and number of teachers depends on your state teacher/student ratio requirements.

Procedure and Questions:

Teacher will explain that all fish swim by using fins. For this lesson, we will not focus on other aspects of fish anatomy.

* Teacher will read the book, *The Rainbow Fish* and emphasize the fins whenever possible.
* Teachers will ask children if they are fish and how do they know.
* Show the children pictures of other animals that can swim and ask them to explain why they are not fish even though they can swim.
* Ask if it is easier to swim like a human or to swim like a fish (there's no right or wrong answer).

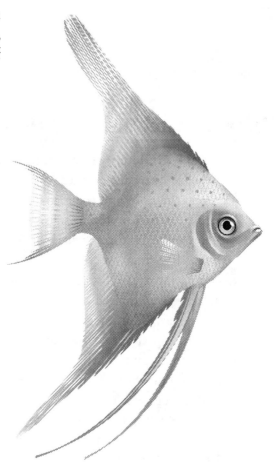

If the classroom has an aquarium this would be a good time to look at the fish and look at their fins. The teacher will ask the children how does the fish use their fins to swim faster or slower.

- Give students the opportunity to be creative and draw their own fish. For this lesson, as long as the drawing has fins, it is a fish.

ACCOMMODATIONS FOR DIVERSE LEARNERS (SPECIAL NEEDS):
All children should be included in this activity regardless of special needs. If a child is unable to lay on the floor to swim, they can swim in whatever position works for them. For a gifted student, teach the difference between the dorsal fins on top of the fish and the pectoral fins on the sides of the fish.

LESSON EXTENSION IDEAS:
Books on the topic of fish should be available in the reading center. The manipulative center can focus on objects found in an aquarium. Art center activities should include pictures of various fish. In the kitchen center, children could have Goldfish crackers for a snack and fish sticks for lunch.

HOW TO CHECK FOR STUDENT UNDERSTANDING:
The teacher will have pictures of various animals that can swim and will ask the students if they are fish. If the children know the animals with fins are fish, they understand the lesson.

EVALUATION OF THE LESSON:
Teachers can evaluate the lesson based on the number of children who could identify whether or not an animal was a fish based on whether or not it had fins.

ACTIVITY 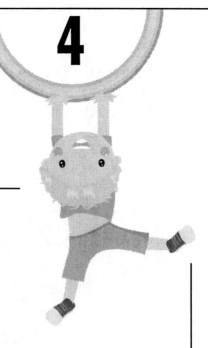 4

AM I A MAMMAL?

GOAL:

To understand life science.

OBJECTIVE:

The children will be able to identify that all mammals are animals that have hair or fur.

Note: For the purpose of this lesson, as long as it has hair or fur, it's a mammal.

Developmental Domain(s) Met:

Physical – Children will go on a nature walk and look for mammals such as squirrels, bunnies, dogs, cats, and other people

Social/Emotional – The children will be put in groups of two and will look at various mammals. They will discuss why an animal is or is not a mammal.

Language and Communication – Children will talk to their partner and to the teacher about why an animal is or is not a mammal.

Cognitive – Children will be exposed to various animals. They will have to determine if it is a mammal by whether or not it has hair or fur.

Creative – After the children view the various types of animals, they will be asked to draw their own mammal (it can be a picture of themselves or any mammal they choose). For the purpose of this lesson, as long as the animal they draw has hair or fur, it's a mammal.

Materials Needed:

* Book – *Is a Camel a Mammal?* By Tish Rabe, Dr. Seuss
* Pictures of mammals such as people, dogs, cats, bunnies, deer, or any other animal that has fur

* Pictures of animals that are not mammals such as birds, insects, fish, reptiles, or any other animal that does not have fur (Supplement#1)
* Paper and crayons

Note: If anyone has a pet mammal they would like to bring in for a demonstration, it will bring the lesson to life (be sure to check for allergies before bringing a mammal to class).

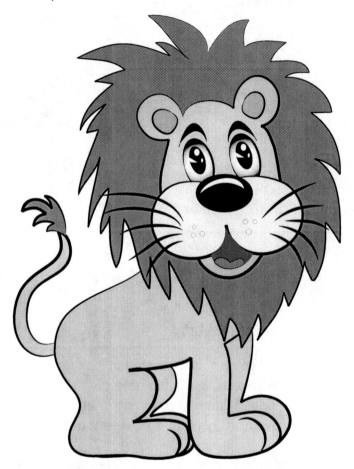

Environment (Indoor/Outdoor, Size of Group):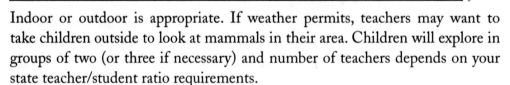

Indoor or outdoor is appropriate. If weather permits, teachers may want to take children outside to look at mammals in their area. Children will explore in groups of two (or three if necessary) and number of teachers depends on your state teacher/student ratio requirements.

Procedure and Questions:

Teacher will explain that all animals that have hair or fur are mammals. The teacher will then explain that not all animals are mammals; for example, birds, fish, and insects are animals but are not mammals. For this lesson, we will not focus on other aspects of mammal anatomy.

- Teacher will read the book, *Is a Camel a Mammal?* and emphasize the hair or fur whenever possible. If a mammal has been brought into the class this would be the time to let the children interact with it in an appropriate fashion.
- Ask children if they are mammals and how do they know.
- Show the children pictures of various animals (mammals and non-mammals) and ask them to explain why each one is or is not a mammal.
- Give children the opportunity to be creative and draw their own mammal. For this lesson, as long as the drawing is an animal that has hair or fur, it is a mammal.

ACCOMMODATIONS FOR DIVERSE LEARNERS (SPECIAL NEEDS): All children should be included in this activity regardless of special needs.

LESSON EXTENSION IDEAS: Books on the topic of mammals should be available in the reading center. The manipulative center should have various animal figures for the children to examine. Art center activities should include pictures of various animals. In the kitchen center, children can have food that comes from mammals, such as any dairy product (check for allergies).

HOW TO CHECK FOR STUDENT UNDERSTANDING: The teacher will have pictures of various animals and will ask the students if they are mammals. The children should know that if the animal has hair or fur, it is a mammal and if it does not have hair or fur, it is not a mammal.

EVALUATION OF THE LESSON: Teachers can evaluate the lesson based on the number of children who could identify whether or not an animal was a mammal based on whether or not it had hair or fur.

ACTIVITY 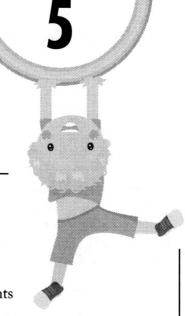 5

AM I A PLANT?

GOAL:

To understand life science.

OBJECTIVE:

The children will be able to identify that all plants grow from the ground.

Note: For the purpose of this lesson, we are only looking at plants that grow from the ground (not aquatic plants or moss).

Developmental Domain(s) Met:

Physical – Children will plant marigold seeds (or any seed the teacher desires) in a Styrofoam cup and must be able to water them on a daily basis.

Social/Emotional – The children will work individually to plant their seeds but will work in groups of two to discuss plants.

Language and Communication – Children will talk to their partner and to the teacher about how to plant their seeds and what plants need to grow.

Cognitive – Children will learn what plants need to grow and will understand the difference between plants and animals.

Creative – The children will draw a fantasy flower garden with their favorite types of plants in it. For the purpose of this lesson, as long as their drawings show plants growing out of the ground, they will be considered plants.

Materials Needed:

* Book: *A Child's Garden: 60 Ideas to Make Any Garden Come Alive for Children* by Molly Dannenmaier
* One Styrofoam cup per child
* One small paper plate per child
* A bag of potting soil

* Water
* Newspaper
* Small Paper Plates
* Seeds (three seeds per child)
* Paper
* Crayons
* The teacher may wish to bring in some potted plants that would be appropriate.
* Pictures of potted plants (Supplement #1)

Environment (Indoor/Outdoor, Size of Group):

Indoor or outdoor is appropriate. Children will go on a nature walk and look for plants. They should be in groups of two (or three if necessary) and number of teachers depends on your state teacher/student ratio requirements.

Procedure and Questions:

* Teacher will read the book and will emphasize that plants grow out of the soil.
* Show the children pictures of plants so they can see that there are many different types of plants but they all grow out of the soil. The teacher will explain that plants grow out of the ground but animals do not.
* Next the children will go on a nature walk and see all the types of plants that grow outside. If any animals are seen, the teacher will emphasize that they are not plants because they do not grow out of the ground.
* When the students return to the classroom, they will plant their seeds.
  1. Give each student a Styrofoam cup and have them put their name on their cup.
  2. The teacher will use a pencil to poke a hole in the bottom of the cup. Explain that the hole will allow excess water to drain so the seed does not drown.
  3. The children will spread newspaper on their work area where they will be planting their seeds.
  4. Use a Styrofoam cup as a scoop to remove the potting soil from the bag and have each child fill their Styrofoam cup approximately three-quarters full with potting soil.
  5. Have children poke three small holes using their fingers in their potting soil. The depth of the hole depends on the directions on the seed packet.
  6. Children will place one seed in each hole and cover them over with potting soil.

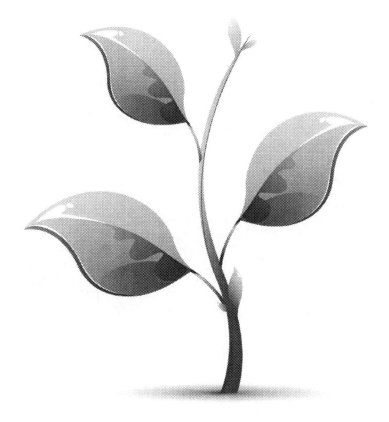

7. Have children place their cups on a paper plate and gently water them until water begins to come out the bottom of the cup.
8. They should place their cups on paper plates in a sunny place, water them daily, and wait for their seeds to germinate.

ACCOMMODATIONS FOR DIVERSE LEARNERS (SPECIAL NEEDS): All children should be included in this activity regardless of special needs.

LESSON EXTENSION IDEAS: Books on the topic of plants should be available in the reading center. Art center activities should include pictures of various plants. In the kitchen center, children should have food that comes from plants and include any type of vegetable or fruit.

HOW TO CHECK FOR STUDENT UNDERSTANDING: The teacher will have pictures of various animals and plants and will ask the students whether each one is a plant. If the children can distinguish that plants grow from the ground and animals do not, they understand the lesson.

EVALUATION OF THE LESSON: Teachers can evaluate the lesson based on the number of children who could identify that plants grow out of the ground and animals do not, and that plants need water, soil and light to grow.

ACTIVITY 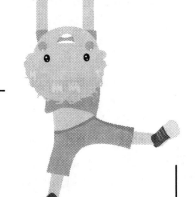 **6**

DON'T BE A LITTERBUG

GOAL:

To understand life and physical sciences.

OBJECTIVE:

The children will be able to understand why litter
is harmful to the environment.

Developmental Domain(s) Met:

Physical – Children will pick up litter in their school environment.

Social/Emotional – The children will work in teams to clean up their school
environment.

Language and Communication – Children will talk to each other and to
the teacher about litter and the importance of not littering.

Cognitive – Children will understand the concepts of why littering is
wasteful and harms the environment.

Creative – Children will draw a picture of a litterbug.

Materials Needed:

* Book: *Cleaning up Litter (Help the Environment)* by Charlotte Gullain
* Examples of recyclable and non-recyclable materials the children will be able
  to collect and identify (see below for examples of materials). The teacher will
  "plant" these items around the school environment for the children to find.
* Paper and crayons
* Two paper grocery bags to collect litter (label recyclable and non-recyclable)

Environment (Indoor/Outdoor, Size of Group):

Inside and outside.

Procedure and Questions:

First the teacher will read the book and explain what litter and recycling are, and the difference between what is recyclable (for example, paper bags, aluminum cans, plastic bottles) and what is not (batteries, paint cans, toothpaste tubes, styrofoam cups).

- Explain what a litterbug is (someone who litters). The teacher will also explain that each of us is responsible for keeping the earth clean and healthy. We each do this by not littering and recycling whenever possible.
- Tell students that they are going to go on a walk around the classroom or the school and pick up any litter they find.
- Children will bring the litter back to a location designated by the teacher.
- After all the litter has been collected, they will go through each piece as a group and decide if it is recyclable or not.
- Have students put the recyclable materials in the paper bag labeled "Recyclable" and the non-recyclable items in the bag labeled "Non-Recyclable." The teacher will explain that there are various ways to handle recyclable and non-recyclable items in the community. The teacher will need to find out how recyclable material is handled in that community.
- After the activity, have the children draw a picture of a litterbug (encourage creativity, the litterbug does not have to be a person, it could be a bug).

ACCOMMODATIONS FOR DIVERSE LEARNERS (SPECIAL NEEDS):
All children should be included in this activity regardless of special needs.

LESSON EXTENSION IDEAS: Books on the environment, litter, and recycling should be available in the reading center. For the art center activity, children can draw pictures of a healthy, clean earth and an unhealthy, littered earth. In the kitchen center, the children should have snacks that only come in recyclable containers or no containers at all.

HOW TO CHECK FOR STUDENT UNDERSTANDING: Engage the children in discussing why littering is bad for the earth. Include reasons such as it's wasteful, it's dangerous (such as toxic or things that could cut your foot), and it's ugly. The teacher will hold up items and ask the children if it is recyclable or not; then ask the students why it is important to not be a litterbug.

EVALUATION OF THE LESSON: Teachers can evaluate the lesson based on the number of children who could correctly answer the questions regarding what items were recyclable or not and why littering is bad for the earth.

ACTIVITY 7

GRAVITY GETS ME DOWN

GOAL:
To understand physical sciences.

OBJECTIVE:
The children will be introduced to the concept that gravity is an invisible force that pulls everything down.

Developmental Domain(s) Met:

Physical – Children will jump up as high as they can and land on their feet. They will slide objects off a table to see that they fall. The teacher will use a book and a ball to illustrate that the ball rolls down the hill and pour water out of a glass to show that water goes down.

Social/Emotional – The children work individually to perform all assigned activities.

Language and Communication – Children will talk to each other and to the teacher about gravity.

Cognitive – Children will understand the concepts of up and down and that even though they can't identify gravity with any of their senses, it's still there.

Creative – Children will draw a picture of gravity pulling something down.

Materials Needed:

* Book – *Up and Down* by Patricia Murphy
* Paper and crayons
* Objects to be dropped to demonstrate gravity
* A ball and a ramp (such as a book)
* A glass, access to a sink and water

Environment (Indoor/Outdoor, Size of Group):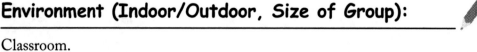

Classroom.

Procedure and Questions:

First the teacher will read the book and explain that gravity is an invisible force that pulls everything toward the earth.

1. Demonstrate several examples of gravity.
   - Hold an object waist high and drop it, explaining that gravity is the force pulling it down.
   - Toss an object gently in the air and explain that it is gravity that stops the object from continuing up into the air and causes it to come down.
   - Gather students around a sink and demonstrate that gravity works on liquids as well as solids. Fill a glass with water and gently pour the water out over the sink, explaining that gravity is what causes the water to fall. Further explain that gravity is what causes the water to go down the drain.
   - Give each child a manipulative and tell them to hold it out waist high and drop it. Explain that gravity caused it to fall down.
   - Then have the children throw the object in the air and explain that gravity stopped it from continuing to go up and caused it to come down.
   - Children will take turns rolling a ball off a ramp explaining that gravity makes the ball fall. Ask: if they put the ball at the bottom of the ramp, why doesn't it roll up?

2. Children experiment if they are stronger than gravity.
   - Students stand up and jump as high and as strong as they can. If they are stronger, they will stay in the air. If gravity is stronger, they will come back down. Which is stronger?

3. Have children draw a picture of something being pulled down by gravity (for example, someone with a parachute or a snowflake).

ACCOMMODATIONS FOR DIVERSE LEARNERS (SPECIAL NEEDS):
All children should be included in this activity regardless of special needs. If you have students with mobility issues, they should be able to participate by dropping objects rather than jumping.

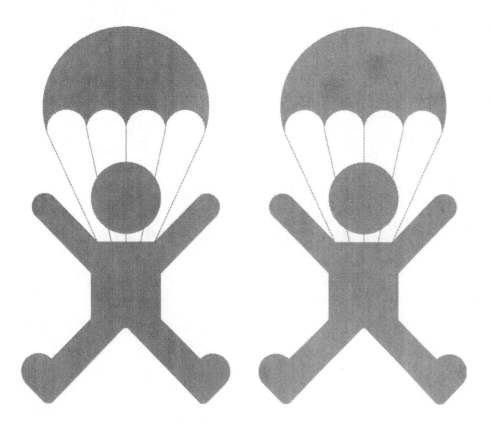

LESSON EXTENSION IDEAS: Books on the topic of gravity should be available in the reading center. Include items the children could drop or bounce in the manipulative center. In the art center activities should include pictures illustrating the effects of gravity.

HOW TO CHECK FOR STUDENT UNDERSTANDING: The teacher will demonstrate the following: hold a manipulative waist high and ask the children what will happen to it when it's let go; put a ball at the base of a ramp and ask why it doesn't roll up; ask the children when they jump, why they don't go up in the sky.

EVALUATION OF THE LESSON: Teachers can evaluate the lesson based on the number of children who could correctly answer the questions about gravity.

ACTIVITY 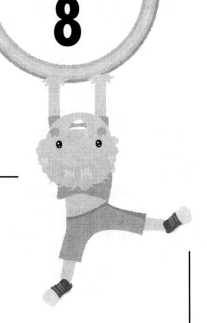 8

I HAVE A HEART

GOAL:

To understand life science.

OBJECTIVE:

The children will identify that all people have
a heart.

Developmental Domain(s) Met:

Physical – Children will put their hand on their chest to feel their heart
beating and use a paper towel roll to hear each other's hearts. Children
will do jumping jacks to make their hearts beat faster.

Social/Emotional – The children will be put in groups of two to listen to
each other's hearts and to understand that when you exercise, your heart
has to beat faster.

Language and Communication – Children will talk to their partner and to
the teacher about hearing their hearts beating.

Cognitive – Children must be able to understand that each heartbeat means
the heart is pumping.

Creative – After the children listen to each other's heartbeat, they will color
a picture of a healthy heart.

Materials Needed:

* Book – *Hear Your Heart* by Paul Showers
* Paper towel tubes
* Copies of Heart Supplement #1
* Crayons

Environment (Indoor/Outdoor, Size of Group):

Classroom. Children will work in groups of two (or three if necessary) and number of teachers depends on your state teacher/student ratio requirements.

Procedure:

The teacher will read the book aloud and allow time for questions. Explain that for this activity the children must be quiet, otherwise they will not be able to hear each other's heartbeat.

- Give one paper towel tube to each group of two students.
- Demonstrate how to use the paper towel tube to hear the partner's heartbeat as is illustrated in the book.
- Teacher will need to work with each group as necessary.
- When everyone has heard their partner's heartbeat, the teacher will explain that the more active your body is, the faster your heart has to beat.
- To illustrate this, instruct one partner in each pair to do jumping jacks (or some other suitable exercise) for 30 seconds. At the end of the exercise, the other partner will use the paper towel tube to listen again to the heartbeat. The children should be able to recognize that the heart is beating faster. Then the children will swap and listen to their partner's heart before and after the exercise.
- Discuss things that will keep your heart healthy. These include things such as eating healthy, getting exercise, and getting plenty of sleep.
- Pass out "I Have A Heart" supplement #1. Ask the children to draw pictures of the things that keep the heart healthy on the supplement page.

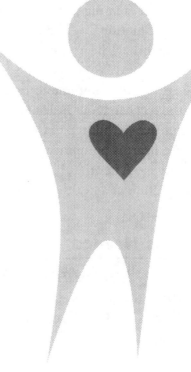

Questions for the Children: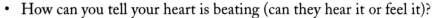

- How can you tell your heart is beating (can they hear it or feel it)?
- Does your heart beat faster or slower when you exercise?
- What are three things a healthy heart needs?

ACCOMMODATIONS FOR DIVERSE LEARNERS (SPECIAL NEEDS):
All children should be included in this activity regardless of special needs. If you have students with mobility issues, the exercise should be appropriate to their needs. For gifted students, have them count the number of heartbeats in 15 seconds.

LESSON EXTENSION IDEAS: Books on the topic of healthy hearts should be available in the reading center. If possible, have a model of the human heart available for children to examine in the manipulative center. Art center activities should include pictures of various exercises to do to keep a heart healthy. In the kitchen center, children can be exposed to heart-healthy foods such as fruit and vegetables.

HOW TO CHECK FOR STUDENT UNDERSTANDING: The teacher will check to see if each student knows how to hear their partner's heart beating using the paper towel tube; if the students understand that their hearts beat faster when they exercise; and if the students can name three things a healthy heart needs.

EVALUATION OF THE LESSON: Teachers can evaluate the lesson based on the number of children who could correctly answer the questions above.

ACTIVITY 9

I HEAR

GOAL:
To understand life science.

OBJECTIVE:
The children will identify objects based on their sense of sound and to understand that anything that blocks our ears will make hearing more difficult.

Developmental Domain(s) Met:

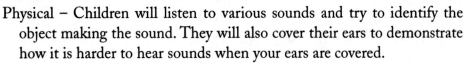

Physical – Children will listen to various sounds and try to identify the object making the sound. They will also cover their ears to demonstrate how it is harder to hear sounds when your ears are covered.

Social/Emotional – Children will work in pairs and compare what they think made the sounds.

Language and Communication – Children will talk to each other and to the teacher about what they are hearing.

Cognitive – Children will need to connect a particular sound with a particular object.

Creative – Children will need to use their imaginations to discern what sound goes with what object.

Materials Needed:

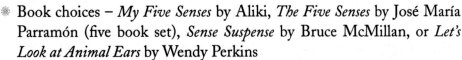

* Book choices – *My Five Senses* by Aliki, *The Five Senses* by José María Parramón (five book set), *Sense Suspense* by Bruce McMillan, or *Let's Look at Animal Ears* by Wendy Perkins
* Computer or tape recorder with recorded sounds such as people laughing, a door closing, an elephant trumpeting, a jet flying, traffic noise, or other sounds that the children would be familiar with

* Pictures of different ears such as human, dog, cat, bunny, and bat ears or any others seen in the book, *Let's Look at Animal Ears*, will be displayed
* Paper and crayons

Environment (Indoor/Outdoor, Size of Group):

Indoors. Children will participate in groups of two (or three if necessary) and number of teachers depends on your state teacher/student ratio requirements.

Procedure and Questions:

The teacher will read a book focusing on the children's sense of hearing.
* Using the computer or tape recorder, play each recorded sound and help the children identify what they think is making the sound.
* Have children cover their ears with their hands and play sounds at the same volume as before.
* Ask the children if it is more difficult to hear when their ears are covered.
* The teacher could show pictures of different kinds of ears based on the animals in the book, then ask why hearing is so important to animals. (For example, animals can hear predators, they can hear prey, and they can hear other sounds like their babies' cry for help.)

ACCOMMODATIONS FOR DIVERSE LEARNERS (SPECIAL NEEDS): All children should be included in this activity regardless of special needs. If you have students with hearing issues, assist them as needed.

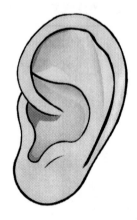

LESSON EXTENSION IDEAS: The art center could have pictures of ears for the children to paint. The kitchen could have samples of food the children can hear such as Rice Crispies, crunchy foods such as carrots, celery, and apples. The book center could have stories about the senses.

HOW TO CHECK FOR STUDENT UNDERSTANDING: The teacher will play different sounds and see if the children can identify objects solely based on the sound it makes. Teacher will also ask children if it is easier to hear the sound when their ears are uncovered and why hearing is so important to humans and other animals.

EVALUATION OF THE LESSON: The teacher can evaluate the lesson based on the number of children who can successfully match an object to it's sound and understand why hearing is important for humans and other animals.

ACTIVITY 10

I SEE

GOAL:

To understand life science.

OBJECTIVE:

The children will differentiate colors (red, blue, green, brown, yellow, and white) based on their sense of sight and to understand that colors are more difficult to see in dim light than in bright.

Developical Domain(s) Met:

Physical – Children will be able to manipulate foods of various colors.

Social/Emotional – Children will work in pairs and compare the color of foods.

Language and Communication – Children will talk to each other and to the teacher about what colors they are seeing.

Cognitive – Children will need to connect the color with the food and other objects.

Creative – Children will need to use their sight to draw a picture incorporating the six colors in the lesson.

Materials Needed:

* Book – *Mouse Paint* by Ellen Stoll Walsh
* Foods of the various colors such as red apples, blueberries, green lettuce, brown potatoes, yellow bananas, white rice
* Items in the colors being discussed (red, blue, green, brown, yellow, and white)
* Brown grocery bags

Environment (Indoor/Outdoor, Size of Group):

Indoors or outdoors and children will participate in groups of two (or three if necessary) and number of teachers depends on your state teacher/student ratio requirements.

Procedure and Questions:

- Teacher will read the book and help the children identify various colors.
- Ask the children to identify one food and its color. Repeat until all foods and all the colors have been identified.
- The teacher will hold up other objects of various colors and see if the children can identify the colors.
- Put an object in the brown grocery bag and have the children look in the bag. Most of the light should be blocked out and the children will determine if it is more difficult to identify the color in the dim light.

ACCOMMODATIONS FOR DIVERSE LEARNERS (SPECIAL NEEDS):
All children should be included in this activity regardless of special needs. If you have students with dexterity issues, they should be assisted as needed. If any child is colorblind, explain that not all people can see various colors.

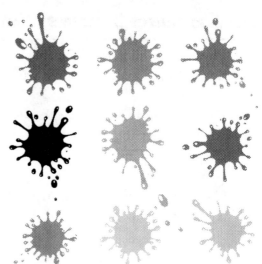

LESSON EXTENSION IDEAS:
The art center could have pictures incorporating many colors. The kitchen area could have samples of the various color foods for the children to taste (check for food allergies prior to having children sample food). Have books on colors in the reading center.

HOW TO CHECK FOR STUDENT
UNDERSTANDING: See if the children can identify the different colors and ask them if it is more difficult to see colors with dim light.

EVALUATION OF THE LESSON: The teacher can evaluate the lesson based on the number of children who can successfully identify colors of various items and could explain that it is more difficult to see colors in dim light.

ACTIVITY 11

I SMELL

GOAL:

To understand life science.

OBJECTIVE:

The children will differentiate objects based on
their sense of smell and to understand that not all animals have the same
kind of nose.

Developmental Domain(s) Met:

Physical – Children will hold cheesecloth-covered cups with different
smelling objects inside to see if they can discern what the object is.

Social/Emotional – Children will work in pairs and compare what they
smell and what they think the object might be.

Language and Communication – Children will talk to each other and to
the teacher about what they are smelling.

Cognitive – Children will need to connect the smell with an object.

Creative – Children will need to use their imaginations to discern what
smell goes with what object. They will also think about different kinds
of noses and what makes each type of nose special.

Materials Needed:

* *The Nose Book* by Al Perkins
* Paper cups
* Cheesecloth cut to fit over the paper cups
* Rubber bands to hold the cheesecloth in place
* Strongly scented items such as a lemon, orange, licorice, peach, onion,
  and tomato (cut each item in half to release the odor)

Environment (Indoor/Outdoor, Size of Group):

Indoor and children will participate in groups of two (or three if necessary) and number of teachers depends on your state teacher/student ratio requirements.

Procedure and Questions:

- Teacher will read the book and help children identify the animals in the book.
- Ask the children why they think different animals have different types of noses and can some animals do more than smell with their nose? For example, an elephant can pick things up with its trunk, an anteater can stick its nose in an anthill, and a dog's sense of smell is better than a human's.
- Ask: If they could have any kind of nose, what would they want and why?
- Give each pair of children a cup containing an object for them to smell. Ask them to identify what the smell is. Do they think it is a good smell or a bad smell and why?

ACCOMMODATIONS FOR DIVERSE LEARNERS (SPECIAL NEEDS): All children should be included in this activity regardless of special needs. If you have students with dexterity issues, hold the cup for them.

LESSON EXTENSION IDEAS: The art center could have pictures of fruit for the children to paint. The kitchen area could have samples of these foods for the children to taste (be sure to check for food allergies). The book center could have stories about the senses.

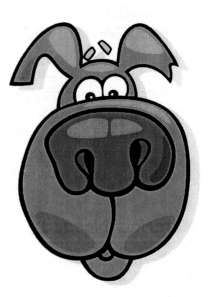

HOW TO CHECK FOR STUDENT UNDERSTANDING: Have pictures of animals with different noses and see if the children can identify which nose goes with each animal. The teacher will determine if the children can identify the various objects based on the object's smell.

EVALUATION OF THE LESSON: The teacher can evaluate the lesson based on the number of children who could identify the nose on the various animals and the number who could identify the object based on the smell.

ACTIVITY 12

I TASTE

GOAL:

To understand life science.

OBJECTIVE:

The children will be able to differentiate foods based
on their sense of taste and to understand that some foods are sweet, some
are sour, and some are salty. Students will also learn about the relationship
between their sense of taste and their sense of smell. They will learn why
food doesn't taste as good when they have a stuffy nose.

Developmental Domain(s) Met:

Physical – Children will hold different foods with different tastes to see if
they can discern what the food is.

Social/Emotional – Children will work in pairs and compare what they
taste and what they think the food might be.

Language and Communication – Children will talk to each other and to
the teacher about what they are tasting.

Cognitive – Children will need to connect the taste with a food and attempt
to predict what a certain food will taste like.

Creative – Children will need to use their imaginations to discern what
taste goes with what food. Children will learn the relationship between
their sense of smell and their sense of taste.

Materials Needed:

* Books to choose from: *My Five Senses* by Aliki, *The Five Senses* by José
  María Parramón (five book set), or *Sense Suspense* by Bruce McMillan
* Sweet tasting food samples such as watermelon, strawberries, or whatever
  sweet fruit is available at the time
* Sour tasting food samples such as lemon, lime, dill pickle

- Salty tasting food such as: pretzel, cracker or potato chip
- Pictures of the foods sampled
- Paper cups
- Water
- Napkins

Environment (Indoor/Outdoor, Size of Group):

Indoors or outdoors and children will participate in groups of two (or three if necessary) and number of teachers depends on your state teacher/student ratio requirements.

Procedure and Questions:

Teacher will read the book and help the children identify various tastes.
Note: Check for food allergies prior to having children sample any food.

- Children will try one food from the sweet category and describe what sweet tastes like.
- Between each tasting, the teacher should have the children drink water to cleanse their palettes.
- Next they will taste something from the sour category to learn what sour tastes like.
- Finally they will taste one food from the salty category to learn what salty tastes like.
- Now the teacher will have the children taste one of the remaining foods from the three categories and see if the children can discern if it is sweet, sour, or salty.
- Repeat this until all foods have been tasted and the teacher is comfortable that the children understand the various tastes.
- Have children discuss their favorite taste and their least favorite taste.
- Next have children taste test a sweet tasting food while they hold their nose closed (this may be awkward for some children so be sure food is cut in small pieces to avoid choking).
- Ask the children if the food tastes the same if they eat it with their nose blocked as it does when they eat and can smell it. There should be less taste when they can't smell the food.
- The teacher might have the children name other foods that might fall into each category.

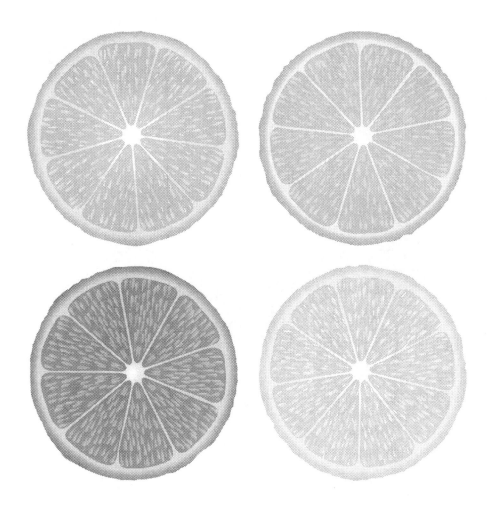

ACCOMMODATIONS FOR DIVERSE LEARNERS (SPECIAL NEEDS): All children should be included in this activity regardless of special needs. If you have students with dexterity issues, they should be assisted as needed.

LESSON EXTENSION IDEAS: The art center could have pictures of fruit for the children to paint. The kitchen area could have samples of these foods for the children to taste. The book center could have stories about tastes.

HOW TO CHECK FOR STUDENT UNDERSTANDING: The teacher will have pictures of the different foods tasted to see if the children can identify if the food is sweet, sour, or salty. The teacher will then ask the children why the food doesn't taste as good when their nose is stuffed up. They should be able to explain that food doesn't taste as good when you can't smell it.

EVALUATION OF THE LESSON: The teacher can evaluate the lesson based on the number of children who can successfully match taste with the different types of food and understand that food doesn't taste as good when you can't smell it.

ACTIVITY 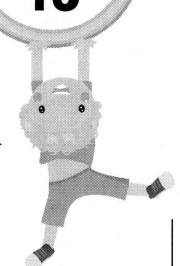 **13**

I TOUCH

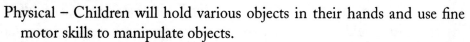

GOAL:

To understand life science.

OBJECTIVE:

The children will be able to identify different
textures based on their sense of touch and to understand that the tips of
their fingers are very sensitive to touch.

Developmental Domain(s) Met:

Physical – Children will hold various objects in their hands and use fine
 motor skills to manipulate objects.

Social/Emotional – Children will work in pairs and discuss with each other
 how they think the various objects feel.

Language and Communication – Children will talk to each other and to
 the teacher about what they are touching. They will have to be able to
 verbalize how an object feels.

Cognitive – Children will need to look at an object and predict how it will feel.

Creative – Children will need to use their imaginations to discuss what the
 objects could be used for based on their texture.

Materials Needed:

- ✳ Book: *Fox in Socks, Bricks and Blocks* by Dr. Seuss
- ✳ Copies of Touch Supplement #1, outline page of various animals (bunny,
 a cat's face, a snake)
- ✳ Fine sandpaper cut into small circles for the cat's tongue
- ✳ Wax paper cut into snake shapes
- ✳ Cotton balls for the bunny tails
- ✳ Glue
- ✳ Crayons

Environment (Indoor/Outdoor, Size of Group):

Indoor and children will participate in groups of two (or three if necessary) and number of teachers depends on your state teacher/student ratio requirements.

Procedure and Questions:

Teacher will read the book and help the children recognize the difference between objects that are soft, rough, and smooth.

- Pass around a cotton ball, a sandpaper piece, and a piece of wax paper to familiarize the children with the three textures.
- Ask the children for examples of things that are soft, rough, and smooth.
- Ask: do you think a bunny tail would be soft, rough, or smooth?
- What do you think a cat's tongue would feel like?
- What do you think a snake would feel like?
- After determining that a bunny tail is soft, the children will glue cotton balls to their bunny picture.
- After determining that a cat's tongue is rough, the children will glue the circle of sandpaper to the cat picture.
- After determining that a snakeskin is smooth, they will glue the wax paper to the picture of the snake.
- The children can color the pictures after the lesson is complete.

ACCOMMODATIONS FOR DIVERSE LEARNERS (SPECIAL NEEDS):
All children should be included in this activity regardless of special needs. If you have students with dexterity issues, they should have the objects held for them.

LESSON EXTENSION IDEAS:
The art center could have pictures of fruit for the children to paint. The kitchen area could have samples of these foods with different textures such as a fuzzy peach, smooth grapes or apples, and a pineapple. The book center could have stories about the senses.

HOW TO CHECK FOR STUDENT UNDERSTANDING:
The teacher will hold up the cotton ball, the sandpaper, and the wax paper and ask the children to identify the different textures. The teacher will determine if the children can identify the various textures based on the object.

EVALUATION OF THE LESSON:
The teacher can evaluate the lesson based on the number of children who could identify the textures based on the objects presented.

ACTIVITY (14)

ADDING BY ONE

GOAL:
To understand basic math concepts.

OBJECTIVE:
The children will be able to add one to the numbers one through five and get the correct number.

Developmental Domain(s) Met:

Physical – Children will use themselves and various manipulatives to see what happens when one is added to the numbers one through five.

Language and Communication – Children will talk to each other and to the teacher about adding one to a number.

Cognitive – Children must be able to count from one to six.

Materials Needed:

* Book: *Maths Made Easy Adding And Taking Away* Preschool Ages 3-5 by Carol Vorderman
* Manipulatives
* Crayons

Environment (Indoor/Outdoor, Size of Group):

Classroom. Children will work as a group.

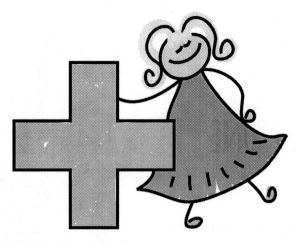

Procedure and Questions:

- Ensure each child can count from one to six.
- Using the book, the teacher will introduce the concept of adding one to a number.
- To demonstrate the concept, have one child come and stand in front of the class.
- Ask the class how many children are standing there.
- Continue adding children to a total of six children, asking how many are standing with each additional child.
- The children will then work in pairs and use manipulatives. The teacher will tell the children to put one manipulative on the table.
- Tell them to add one manipulative and give the resulting number.
- The children will continue adding one manipulative at a time until they have a total of six.
- The teacher may repeat this as often as needed with different manipulatives.

ACCOMMODATIONS FOR DIVERSE LEARNERS (SPECIAL NEEDS):
All children should be included in this activity regardless of special needs.

LESSON EXTENSION IDEAS: Books on the topic of numbers should be available in the reading center. In the manipulative center, the focus should be on counting items from one to six. In the kitchen center snacks could be distributed by adding one more to whatever the children already have.

HOW TO CHECK FOR STUDENT UNDERSTANDING: The children will give a number between one and five and asked what number will result if they add one more to that number. The teacher will determine if the children can answer correctly.

EVALUATION OF THE LESSON: Teachers can evaluate the lesson based on the number of children who can correctly add one to the numbers one to five.

ACTIVITY 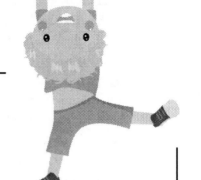 15

CINNAMON APPLE SLICES

GOAL:

To understand basic math concepts.

OBJECTIVE:

The children will be able to follow directions to make an edible treat.

Developmental Domain(s) Met:

Physical – Children will manipulate cooking ingredients.

Language and Communication – Children will talk to each other and to the teacher about following the procedures to make apple treats.

Cognitive – Children must be able to measure ingredients and follow directions.

Materials Needed:

* One apple for every two children
* Cinnamon
* Sugar
* Plastic sandwich bags
* Measuring spoons
* Paper plates
* Wet Ones or a sink for washing hands
* Bowls for cinnamon and sugar

Environment (Indoor/Outdoor, Size of Group):

Classroom. Children will work individually.

Procedure and Questions:

Before the activity, the teacher will slice each apple into eight pieces and remove the core. Be sure to check for food allergies.

- Have the children wash their hands.
- Give each child one sandwich bag and one paper plate with four apple slices on it. Tell the children not to eat the apple slices yet.
- Each child will take their baggie up to the teacher for assistance in measuring one tablespoon of sugar and one-half teaspoon of cinnamon into the baggie, and seal their baggies with help from the teacher if necessary.
- Tell children to shake their baggie to mix the sugar and cinnamon.
- Instruct them to reopen their baggie, being careful not to spill the sugar and cinnamon, and place the four apple slices inside.
- Have children reseal their baggie and shake the baggie to coat the apples with the sugar and cinnamon mixture.
- The children may then open their baggies and enjoy the treats they've made.

Ask the children:

- Why do you need to be sure your baggie is sealed before you shake it?
- How much sugar and how much cinnamon did you add to the baggie?
- How many slices of apple did you add to the baggie?
- Why did we mix the cinnamon and sugar before adding the apples?

ACCOMMODATIONS FOR DIVERSE LEARNERS (SPECIAL NEEDS): All children should be included in this activity regardless of special needs.

LESSON EXTENSION IDEAS: Books on the topic of cooking should be available in the reading center. In the manipulative center, the focus should be on cooking items. This will be the snack for the day.

HOW TO CHECK FOR STUDENT UNDERSTANDING: The teacher will see if the children can follow directions and answer the questions asked.

EVALUATION OF THE LESSON: Teachers can evaluate the lesson based on the number of children who can follow the directions and correctly answer the questions.

ACTIVITY 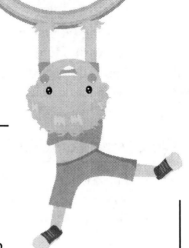 16

EVEN OR ODD

GOAL:
To understand basic math concepts.

OBJECTIVE:
The children will be able to tell whether a group of objects is even or odd.

Developmental Domain(s) Met:

Physical – Children will use a crayon and circle objects in groups of two.

Language and Communication – Children will talk to each other and to the teacher about the whether a group is even or odd.

Cognitive – Children must be able to place objects into groups of two to decide if something is even or odd. Children will understand that if one item is left out, then it is an odd number of objects. If the objects can be put in groups of two, it is even.

Materials Needed:

* Book: *Scholastic Reader Level 3: Even Steven and Odd Todd* by Kathryn Cristaldi and Henry Morehouse
* Even/Odd Supplement #1
* Crayons

Environment (Indoor/Outdoor, Size of Group):

Classroom. Children will work individually.

Procedure:

The teacher will explain that all even numbers can be put in groups of two. If it is an odd number, one object will always be left out.

- Teacher will demonstrate by drawing an even number of objects and drawing circles around the groups of two. The teacher will then show that with odd numbers, one object will always be left over.
- The children will use the "Even/Odd Supplement #1" and draw a circle around any groups of items that are even.

Questions for Children:

- The teacher will hold up various numbers of fingers or other manipulatives and ask the children if it is even or odd.
- Teacher will then ask the children how they know if it is even or odd?

ACCOMMODATIONS FOR DIVERSE LEARNERS (SPECIAL NEEDS): All children should be included in this activity regardless of special needs.

LESSON EXTENSION IDEAS: Books on the topic of numbers should be available in the reading center. In the manipulative center, the focus should be on counting even and odd groups of items. In the kitchen center snacks could be distributed in groups of even or odd. Children will be asked to identify if they received an even or odd snack.

HOW TO CHECK FOR STUDENT UNDERSTANDING: The teacher will give each child a group of items and have them determine if it is even or odd. Teacher will determine if the children can check-off the correct response on the "Even/Odd Supplement #1."

EVALUATION OF THE LESSON: Teachers can evaluate the lesson based on the number of children who can correctly answer if a group of objects is even or odd.

ACTIVITY 17

MARSHMALLOW STRUCTURES

GOAL:

To expose children to basic concepts of geometry.

OBJECTIVE:

The children will be given the information needed
to build shapes and three-dimensional structures using marshmallows
and toothpicks.

Developmental Domain(s) Met:

Physical – Fine motor; manipulating small materials.
Cognitive – Shapes, dimension and support concepts, trial and error.
Creative – Visualization and confinement-free construction.

Materials Needed:

* Miniature marshmallows (15 to 20 per child)
* Round wood toothpicks (15 to 20 per child)
* Paper towels (for working surface)

Environment (Indoor/Outdoor, Size of Group):

Indoor, group size 8 to 12 (this activity is best with 4-year-olds and older).

Procedure:

- Show children photos of various buildings.
- Show children pictures of geometric shapes.
- Pass around different shapes for the children to hold.
- Discuss the properties of each shape.

- Have each child wash their hands before they begin.
- Show children toothpicks and marshmallows, explaining safety practices with the toothpicks.
- Model building different shapes with the toothpicks and marshmallows.
- Model how to attach the shapes to each other by pushing the toothpicks into the marshmallows to create two- and three-dimensional structures.
- Explain that each child will make their own shapes and structures and once they have made four shapes and at least one structure for you to see, then they will be able to eat their marshmallows. (Check for allergies before letting children eat.)

Questions for Children:

- What makes each shape different from the others?
- Open-ended questions about what holds up homes and other buildings.

LESSON EXTENSION IDEAS:
- Provide a math shape center with manipulatives and puzzles
- Play Twister!

HOW TO CHECK FOR STUDENT UNDERSTANDING: As you ask questions, determine which children recognize the shapes, which children can explain the differences between the shapes, and which children can build a three-dimensional structure.

ACCOMMODATIONS FOR DIVERSE LEARNERS (SPECIAL NEEDS): Work with children one-on-one to help them create shapes. Use pretzel sticks and large marshmallows. Have three-dimensional shapes for the children to feel and explore.

EVALUATION OF THE LESSON: The teacher will evaluate the activity based on the level of understanding shown by the children and their enjoyment of the activity.

ACTIVITY 18

MITTEN MATCHING

GOAL:

To expose children to the concept of patterns and mirror image.

OBJECTIVE:

The children will design a pattern on a pair of paper mittens.

Developmental Domain(s) Met:

Physical – Fine motor: coloring.
Language and Communication – Listening to a story.
Cognitive – Drawing and matching patterns; symmetry.
Creative – Artistic unique design.

Materials Needed:

* Book – *The Mitten* by Jan Brett
* One pair of construction paper mittens per child
* Markers or crayons
* Hot cocoa and cups, optional

Environment (Indoor/Outdoor, Size of Group):

Indoor, group size 8 to 12 (this activity is best with 4-year-olds and older).

Procedure and Questions:

- Read the story
- Ask children what they think will happen next; let the children look for clues. (Jan Brett stories have clues about what is coming next before you turn the page.)
- Show the children a pair of plain white construction paper mittens.
- Discuss patterns and symmetry.
- Using markers or crayons, create a pattern on your mittens matching the design on each.
- Give each child a pair of mittens to create their own design on.
- Put all of the finished mittens in a pile and play a game of mitten matching.

LESSON EXTENSION IDEAS:
- Prepare hot chocolate for the children to drink while making their mittens, checking for allergies.
- Give the children inexpensive paper plates to use for "ice skating," tie the mittens together using a hole punch and yarn for them to wear around their necks while skating!
- Have children stuff three white trash bags with newspaper when they complete their mittens. Later turn the stuffed bags into a snowman.

HOW TO CHECK FOR STUDENT UNDERSTANDING: Observe each child's ability to anticipate what is going to happen next in the story. Observe and record each child's ability to make a pattern and repeat it symmetrically on each mitten.

ACCOMMODATIONS FOR DIVERSE LEARNERS (SPECIAL NEEDS):
Some children may be able to cut out their own mitten pattern. Provide examples of patterns for children.

EVALUATION OF THE LESSON: The teacher will evaluate the lesson based on the number of children that are able to anticipate the story, understand patterns, and create patterns.

ACTIVITY 19

MORE OR LESS

GOAL:

To understand basic math concepts.

OBJECTIVE:

The children will identify whether a manipulated number of objects is more or less than the original number of objects.

Developmental Domain(s) Met:

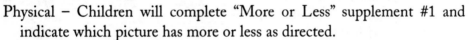

Physical – Children will complete "More or Less" supplement #1 and indicate which picture has more or less as directed.

Language and Communication – Children will talk to each other and to the teacher about numbers of objects and whether they are more or less than the original number.

Cognitive – Children must be able to understand that when you add an object, it is more and when you take one away, it is less.

Materials Needed:

* Book: *A Million Fish...More or Less*, by Patricia McKissack
* "More or Less" Supplement #1
* Crayons

Environment (Indoor/Outdoor, Size of Group):

Classroom. Children will work individually and in groups.

Procedure:

- The teacher will explain the concept of more or less.
- Explain that more is a greater number of something and less is smaller number.
- Use manipulatives to demonstrate the number of objects and identify more or less.
- Teacher will demonstrate with some pictures, diagrams, and any manipulatives to show more or less.
- The children will use the "More or Less" supplement #1 to indicate their understanding of the concept.

Questions for Children:

- The teacher will present various manipulatives, diagrams, and pictures to see if the children can identify more or less.
- Ask the children how they know if it is a pattern more or less.

ACCOMMODATIONS FOR DIVERSE LEARNERS (SPECIAL NEEDS): All children should be included in this activity regardless of special needs.

LESSON EXTENSION IDEAS: Books on the topic of more or less should be available in the reading center. In the manipulative center, the focus should be on categorizing objects and identifying more or less.

HOW TO CHECK FOR STUDENT UNDERSTANDING: The teacher will give each child a "More or Less" supplement #1 and see if the children can identify more or less. Teacher will determine if the children understand the concept based on the sheet and their interaction with other students.

EVALUATION OF THE LESSON: Teachers can evaluate the lesson based on the number of children who can correctly identify more or less on their supplement.

ACTIVITY 20

PATTERNS

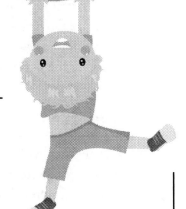

GOAL:

To understand basic math concepts.

OBJECTIVE:

The children will identify patterns and be able to continue a pattern that has already been started.

Developmental Domain(s) Met:

Physical – Children will use a crayon to continue patterns.

Language and Communication – Children will talk to each other and to the teacher about patterns.

Cognitive – Children must be able to continue a pattern that has been started.

Materials Needed:

* Book: *Bees, Snails, & Peacock Tails: Patterns & Shapes* by Betsy Franco & Steve Jenkins
* Pattern Supplement #1
* Crayons

Environment (Indoor/Outdoor, Size of Group):

Classroom. Children will work individually.

Procedure:

- The teacher will explain what a pattern is and how to follow it.
- Explain that a pattern is a repeating sequence of objects, that could be based on shape, color, or other categories.
- Demonstrate some simple patterns for example; square, circle, square, circle, or, red circle, yellow circle, or, dog, house, dog, house.
- The children will use the "Pattern Supplement #1" to identify and continue the patterns that have been started.

Questions for Children:

- The teacher will present various patterns and see if the children can identify the pattern and then continue the pattern.
- Ask the children how they know if it is a pattern based on whether it repeats.

ACCOMMODATIONS FOR DIVERSE LEARNERS (SPECIAL NEEDS): All children should be included in this activity regardless of special needs.

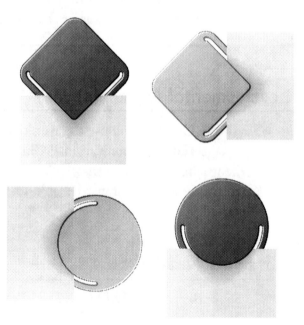

LESSON EXTENSION IDEAS: Books on the topic of pattern should be available in the reading center. In the manipulative center, the focus should be on making patterns out of objects and continuing the patterns.

HOW TO CHECK FOR STUDENT UNDERSTANDING: The teacher will give each child a pattern sheet and see if they can continue the pattern. Teacher will determine if the children understand what a pattern is and how to continue a pattern that has been started.

EVALUATION OF THE LESSON: Teachers can evaluate the lesson based on the number of children who can correctly identify and continue patterns.

ACTIVITY 21

SHAPE-O-SAURUS

GOAL:
To expose children to shapes and colors.

OBJECTIVE:
The children will be given construction paper shapes in a variety of colors to use in creating a dinosaur picture.

Developmental Domain(s) Met:

Physical – Fine motor; cutting, gluing, coloring.
Cognitive – Names of colors and shapes.
Creative – Interpretation of what a dinosaur would look like.

Materials Needed:

* Books about dinosaurs
* Construction paper shapes (depending on the age, these can be already cut out or the children can cut them out)
* One 9 x 12 sheet of black construction paper per child
* Glue
* Oil pastels
* Scissors (depending on the age)

Environment (Indoor/Outdoor, Size of Group):

Indoor, group size 8 to 12.

Procedure:

- Read a fun book about dinosaurs.
- Show the children colorful cut out circles, squares, triangles, and ovals and rectangles in different lengths.
- Discuss the properties of each shape and compare the shapes.
- Model placing the colorful shapes on a sheet of 9 x 12 black construction paper using the pieces to create a dinosaur (e.g., triangles make great spike plates on necks and tails)
- Show the students that once they are happy with what their dinosaur looks like, they can glue down the pieces.
- Use the oil pastels to color the area around the dinosaur creating plants, water, mountains, and/or volcanoes. (You can revisit the book to help the children get ideas for their scenery.)
- Let each child write the name of their dinosaur on the artwork using their name for the first part (e.g., "Daniel-o-saurus" or "Megan-o-saurus").

Questions for Children:

- What shapes have you used?
- What is different about each shape?
- What colors have you used?

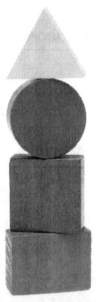

LESSON EXTENSION IDEAS:
- Play "find a shape" or "I spy" and have the children find shapes in common materials in the classroom.
- Create a class "box-o-saurus" having the children bring in boxes, paint them, and build a large three-dimensional dinosaur.

HOW TO CHECK FOR STUDENT UNDERSTANDING:
Ask the children the names of the colors they chose, the names of the shapes they chose, and the differences between the shapes.

ACCOMMODATIONS FOR DIVERSE LEARNERS (SPECIAL NEEDS):
Have shapes already cut out for the children. Have plastic dinosaurs and shapes for the children to feel and look at while creating their art. Have a shape and color chart on the table or surface where the child is working.

EVALUATION OF THE LESSON:
The teacher will evaluate the activity based on the level of understanding and how many children could correctly answer questions about the shapes and colors.

ACTIVITY 22

SHAPES

GOAL:

To understand basic math concepts.

OBJECTIVE:

The children will identify a circle, a triangle, and
a square, and to be able to tell how many sides and corners each shape has.

Developmental Domain(s) Met:

Physical – Children will use a crayon to draw a circle, a triangle, and a square.

Language and Communication – Children will talk to each other and to the teacher about circles, triangles, and squares.

Cognitive – Children must be able to identify the shape and tell how many sides and corners each shape has.

Materials Needed:

* Book: *Bees, Snails, & Peacock Tails: Patterns & Shapes* by Betsy Franco & Steve Jenkins
* Shape Supplement #1
* Crayons
* Blank paper

Environment (Indoor/Outdoor, Size of Group):

Classroom. Children will work individually.

Procedure:

- The teacher will explain that a square has four equal sides and four corners, a triangle has three sides and three corners, and a circle has one line and no corners.
- Demonstrate that the size doesn't matter; for example, a small square, a big triangle, a small circle by presenting pictures of varying sizes.
- Using the "Shape Supplement #1," the teacher will point to the square and ask the children what it is, how many sides it has, and how many corners it has.
- Repeat this with the circle and the triangle until you are comfortable that the children understand the concepts.
- Using "Shape Supplement #1" as a reference, ask the children to use a separate sheet to draw a big and little circle, a big and little triangle, and a big and little square.

Questions for Children:

- Present a circle, a triangle, and a square and see if the children can identify them.
- Ask the children how many sides each shape has and how many corners each shape has.

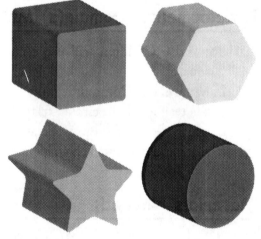

ACCOMMODATIONS FOR DIVERSE LEARNERS (SPECIAL NEEDS): All children should be included in this activity regardless of special needs.

LESSON EXTENSION IDEAS: Books on the topic of shapes should be available in the reading center. In the manipulative center, the focus should be on circles, triangles, and squares.

HOW TO CHECK FOR STUDENT UNDERSTANDING: The teacher will ask each child to draw a circle, a triangle, and a square; then ask each child how many sides and corners each of those shapes has.

EVALUATION OF THE LESSON: Teachers can evaluate the lesson based on the number of children who can correctly identify each shape and can tell how many sides and corners each shape has.

ACTIVITY 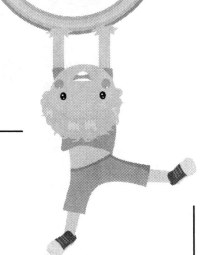 23

TWO OF A KIND

GOAL:

To understand basic math concepts.

OBJECTIVE:

The children will identify pairs of items.

Developmental Domain(s) Met:

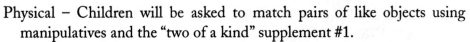

Physical – Children will be asked to match pairs of like objects using manipulatives and the "two of a kind" supplement #1.

Language and Communication – Children will talk to each other and to the teacher about what makes two objects a pair.

Cognitive – Children will understand the concept of two of a kind makes a pair.

Creative – Children will draw a picture of their favorite things in pairs.

Materials Needed:

* "Two of a Kind" Supplement #1
* Paper and crayons
* Pairs of manipulatives to illustrate the concept of "two of a kind"

Environment (Indoor/Outdoor, Size of Group):

Classroom

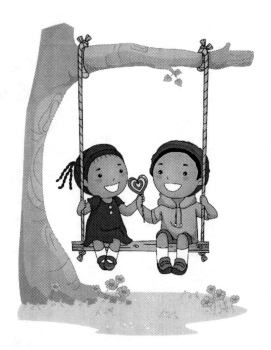

Procedure and Questions:

- Explain that a pair means "two of a kind" and then demonstrate pairs using manipulatives.
- The teacher will explain "Two of a Kind" supplement #1 and have the children complete it.
- Have the children draw a pair of their favorite things.
- Ask: What makes something a pair?
- Explain that two of the same things make it a pair.
- Hold up one object and ask if it is a pair.
- Hold up three identical objects and ask if it's a pair.
- Then hold up two identical objects and ask if it is a pair.

ACCOMMODATIONS FOR DIVERSE LEARNERS (SPECIAL NEEDS): All children should be included in this activity regardless of special needs.

LESSON EXTENSION IDEAS: Two of a kind items should be available in the manipulative center. In the kitchen area children could make snacks that included two of each item (pretzels, Goldfish).

HOW TO CHECK FOR STUDENT UNDERSTANDING: The teacher will hold up manipulatives and ask if they are a pair. Check the Resource Pages to see if the children were able to identify the pairs correctly.

EVALUATION OF THE LESSON: Teachers can evaluate the lesson based on the number of children who could correctly identify pairs and completed their resource pages.

ACTIVITY 24

THE VERY HANDY CATERPILLAR

GOAL:

To expose children to the life cycle of the butterfly

OBJECTIVE:

The children will read "The Very Hungry Caterpillar" by Eric Carle and create a caterpillar painting

Developmental Domain(s) Met:

Physical – Fine motor; painting
Language and Communication – Children discuss the life cycle of the butterfly, habitats and protecting butterflies
Creative – Each caterpillar will be unique to the child

Materials Needed:

* The book "The Very Hungry Caterpillar" by Eric Carle
* Photos of eggs, caterpillars, chrysalis, Monarch butterflies, milkweed plants
* Children's finger paint (green, black, red, yellow)
* White heavy construction paper
* Paintbrushes

Environment (Indoor/Outdoor, Size of Group):

Indoor or outdoor at tables
Group size 6 - 8 (this activity is best with ages 3-5)

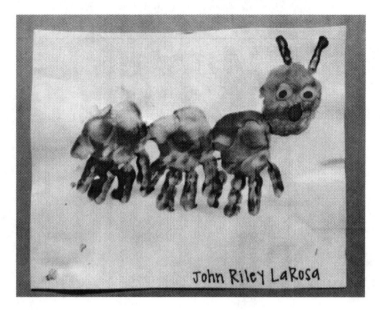

John Riley LaRosa

Procedure and Questions:

Note – This activity can be part of a thematic study of butterflies, the life cycle and habitats.

Read the story "The Very Hungry Caterpillar" to the children

Ask open-ended questions that help the children discuss facts about caterpillars and the life cycle of butterflies. Include questions about how an egg turns into caterpillar, forms a chrysalis and then becomes a butterfly.

Explain that each child is going to make their own caterpillar.

Model the project in front of the children.
1. Paint the palm of the child's hand with green paint and their fingers (except for the thumb) with brown paint. Have the child put their handprint on the paper four times (adding more paint to their hand before doing each handprint). Make the body and legs of the caterpillar.
2. Paint the palm of the child's hand with red paint to make the head of the caterpillar.
3. After the paint dries add the details (antennae, eyes and nose).

LESSON EXTENSION IDEAS: Create a butterfly habitat in your classroom (aquarium, caterpillar, leaves, a stick for the caterpillar to form a chrysalis on). Discuss the migration of Monarch butterflies and take a fieldtrip to observe them. Make cutouts of butterflies and have the children color them like Monarch butterflies.

HOW TO CHECK FOR STUDENT UNDERSTANDING: Understanding can be checked by responses to open-ended questions regarding lifecycles of butterflies, caterpillars, eggs, chrysalis and habitats.

ACCOMMODATIONS FOR DIVERSE LEARNERS (SPECIAL NEEDS): Provide one-on-one guidance.

EVALUATION OF THE LESSON: You will observe the different ability levels of the children and determine the number of teachers needed to assist with the activity.

Section 3

PHYSICAL DEVELOPMENT, HEALTH, AND SOCIAL SCIENCE

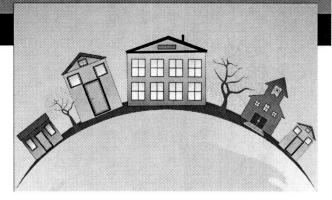

There is a major movement nationwide to make sure the children of tomorrow are in better health and physical shape than those of today. There is renewed emphasis on healthy food choices, both in childcare centers and school cafeterias. The use of physical exercise in the childcare setting is also being stressed on a daily basis. These lesson plans will promote healthy eating habits as well as large and small motor development activities that will continue to keep children active.

In the Social Science section of this resource manual, a combination of home, community, and school interactive lesson plans are introduced providing parent involvement, development of social and emotional skills, and the building of self-esteem. The plans provide for continuity of the children's social and emotional lives from the classroom to the home environment.

All the lesson plans have a "hands-on" approach to learning, and encourage creativity, exploration, and discovery. Children need to experience a healthy lifestyle in order to continue that lifestyle when they are older. The lessons encourage social, emotional, and physical health, and start children on the path to a healthy life.

Added emphasis is placed on safety, especially on the playground. A lesson plan on "Safe Play" encourages young children to participate in creating safety rules for the playground, helping them participate in the safe play. This gives the children ownership of their learning and playing environment.

ACTIVITY 1

APPLE TASTING

GOAL:

To use the five senses while tasting various types of apples.

OBJECTIVE:

The children will be able to identify the five senses
and use them while tasting different types of apples.

Developmental Domain(s) Met:

Language and Communication – The children will be able to communicate
which apples he/she likes and dislikes.

Cognitive – The children will be able to count the apples and identify the
colors of the apples.

Creative – The children will draw a picture of their favorite type of apple.

Materials Needed:

* Various types of apples, such as fresh (red, yellow, green), dried, applesauce,
  apple juice. A small amount of each apple type for each child.
* Paper plates
* Markers or paint
* Drawing paper for each child

Environment (Indoor/Outdoor, Size of Group):

Any size group, seated at tables in the classroom.

Procedure:

Before the lesson, prepare a small amount of each apple type on a paper plate for each child. Check for children with food allergies.

- Begin the lesson by writing the word Apple on the board.
- The children will read the word and discuss various types of apples.
- Write the five senses on the board; Hearing, sight, touch, smell, and taste; explaining each one.
- Pass out the apple plates and have each child taste the apples one at a time as a group. The students will describe how the apple tastes, smells, and feels.
- After all of the apples are eaten, have the children draw or paint a picture of their favorite apple and write the word "apple" if they are able to.

Questions for Children:

- What type of apple is your favorite?
- What did the apples taste, feel, and smell like?
- How many apple types did you try?

LESSON EXTENSION IDEAS: The children will draw or paint a picture of their favorite type of apple. The teacher will sing the song B-I-N-G-O, changing the letters to A-P-P-L-E.

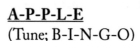

A-P-P-L-E
(Tune; B-I-N-G-O)

There's a fruit that's good for you and apple is its name-O.
A-P-P-L-E, A-P-P-L-E, A-P-P-L-E,
And apple is its name-O!

HOW TO CHECK FOR STUDENT UNDERSTANDING: The teacher will take note of which children participated in the activity and if the children were able to draw a picture of their favorite apple.

ACCOMMODATIONS FOR DIVERSE LEARNERS (SPECIAL NEEDS): Children with special needs may need help understanding the five senses and drawing the picture.

EVALUATION OF THE LESSON: The teacher will evaluate the lesson based on the children's enjoyment, understanding, and participation.

ACTIVITY 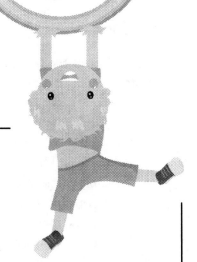 2

CAFÉ PRE-K

GOAL:

To understand healthy eating habits.

OBJECTIVE:

The children will be able to order healthy meals when eating out.

Developmental Domain(s) Met:

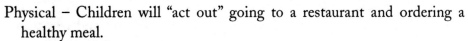

Physical – Children will "act out" going to a restaurant and ordering a healthy meal.

Social/Emotional – Children will take on various roles such as cook, hostess, customer, server, and dishwasher.

Language and Communication – Children will talk to each other and to the teacher about going to a restaurant and ordering a healthy meal.

Cognitive – Children must be able to understand that they have choices when they go out to eat and there are healthy and unhealthy choices for food.

Creative – Children will use their imaginations to create a restaurant environment and take on various character's roles.

Materials Needed:

* Book – *The Berenstain Bears Go Out to Eat* by Jan and Mike Berenstain
* Tables
* Tablecloths
* Chairs
* Notepad and pencil (to take orders)
* Healthy food choices
* Paper plates
* Napkins
* Dramatic play clothes (cook, server, dishwasher, guests)

Environment (Indoor/Outdoor, Size of Group):

Classroom

Procedure:

Teacher will read the book in the large group and introduce the topic of going to a restaurant and ask the students questions about their favorite restaurants.

- Explain that for this activity the children must work as a team. They will need to create a restaurant, take on various roles and decide what food they will serve for a healthy meal.
- Help the children set up the classroom so it looks like a restaurant.
- Teacher will need to work with the group as necessary. Each student will be responsible for some aspect of setting up the restaurant, preparing and serving the food.
- Help the children create a menu with healthy meal choices.
- The children will take on their character's role and act out the restaurant experience.

Questions for the Children:

- What role did you play at the restaurant?
- What meal choices did you have at the restaurant and why were those healthy?
- What is your favorite healthy food choice and why?

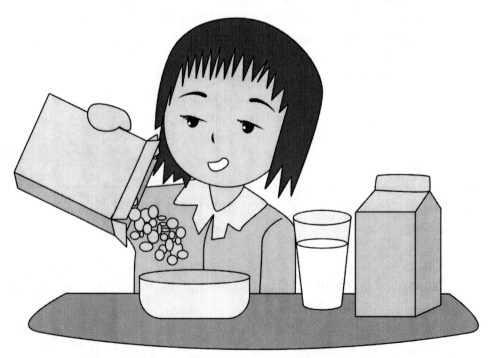

ACCOMMODATIONS FOR DIVERSE LEARNERS (SPECIAL NEEDS):
All children should be included in this activity regardless of special needs.

LESSON EXTENSION IDEAS: Books on the topic of healthy eating choices
should be available in the reading center. In the manipulative center, restaurant items such as fruits and vegetables should be available for children to examine. In the art center activities should include pictures of various types of food.

HOW TO CHECK FOR STUDENT UNDERSTANDING: The teacher will
check to see if each student knows how to order a healthy meal when they go out to a restaurant. Ask the children to give examples of healthy meals they can have when they go out to eat.

EVALUATION OF THE LESSON:
Teachers can evaluate the lesson based on the number of children who could correctly answer the questions above.

ACTIVITY **3**

COMMUNITY HELPERS FAIR

GOAL:

To promote community spirit and interaction in childcare/preschool environments.

OBJECTIVE:

The children will create a "community helpers" fair featuring various occupations dealing with people.

Developmental Domain(s) Met:

Physical – Students will participate in physical activities related to certain occupations and their job requirements. For example, firefighters must be able to lift weights.

Social/Emotional – Children will interact with parents and other community helpers.

Language and Communication – Children will use descriptive words to talk about the various community helpers and what they do.

Cognitive – Children will understand that people perform different jobs in the community that help us. Books will be used to illustrate various occupations and what they do to help others.

Creative - Children will be asked to dress up as the occupation they would like to be. A dress-up corner will provide props for various occupations.

Materials Needed:

* Book: *Community Helpers from A to Z* by Bobbie Kalman
* Invitations for guests
* Food
* Tables
* Chairs
* Costumes/props
* Programs

Environment (Indoor/Outdoor, Size of Group):

Classroom

Procedure:

The teacher will introduce the concept of a "Community Helpers Fair" to the children in the group setting.

- Explain that it takes many helpers to keep a community healthy and safe. Ask the children who keeps them safe and healthy.
- Invitations will be made for all the possible attendees such as police, firefighters, EMTs, nurses, doctors, grocers, construction workers, military, postal workers, and landscapers.
- Involve the children in planning the event. Ask the children if any of their parents are involved in this type of work and if they would like to come to the Community Helpers Fair.
- Talk about possible times, what will be served, if they would like to dress up as their favorite occupation (they can stand next to that person as they are introduced) and if they would like to be greeters, hostesses, and servers.
- Explain that Community Helpers will come to class and talk about what they do for their jobs and how they keep the community safe and healthy.

Questions for the Children:

- Who are community helpers?
- What does each of them do?
- Why are community helpers important?
- Which community helper would you want to be?

Questions to Ask the Guests at the Fair:

- What is your job?
- Do you like your job? Why?
- What will children need to learn in school if they are going to do your job?

LESSON EXTENSION IDEAS: Children will interact with the guests at the fair while they enjoy food and drink. See if a child or a group would be allowed to actually go to the fire station and sit in a truck, or visit the post office, police station, or sit in a police car.

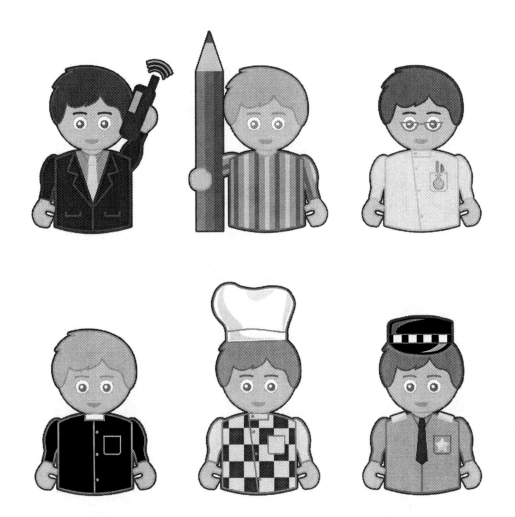

HOW TO CHECK FOR STUDENT UNDERSTANDING: Children will have group time after the event to share the duties and expectations of community helpers as well as tell why they might want to be a certain one.

ACCOMMODATIONS FOR DIVERSE LEARNERS (SPECIAL NEEDS): Consider inviting a social worker or someone who works with special needs children to be a part of this group, for example, a speech therapist.

EVALUATION OF THE LESSON: Assessment—After the fair is over children will provide feedback on what worked and what didn't as well as suggestions for the next event. Teacher will evaluate the lesson based on the number of children who can explain what a Community Helper is, how they keep the community safe and healthy, and what they need to learn in school for those jobs.

ACTIVITY 4

CUTTING POOL CENTER

GOAL:
To give children the opportunity to develop fine motor cutting skills.

OBJECTIVE:
The children will be provided with scissors to use in free cutting and line cutting activities in a contained space.

Developmental Domain(s) Met:

Physical – Fine motor: manipulating scissors and paper.
Social/Emotional – Practicing a skill with a small group.
Creative – Process cutting.

Materials Needed:

* A hard plastic child size swimming pool (open with no slide)
* Scrap construction paper
* Paper with various lines, patterns, shapes, and pictures
* Children's scissors

Environment (Indoor/Outdoor, Size of Group):

Indoor or outdoor. Group size 2 to 3 (this activity is best with 4-year-olds and older).

Procedure:

* Put cutting paper in the hard plastic pool, placing the pool in the corner of the classroom or outside.
* Demonstrate proper grip of scissors (thumb up).

- Demonstrate how to hold and turn paper as you cut (thumb up).
- Demonstrate free form cutting and cutting on lines.
- Monitor children during their time in the cutting pool.

Questions for Children:

- Can you show me the right way to hold your scissors?
- What is not okay to use your scissors on? (Hair, clothes, friends.)
- What are you allowed to cut? (Only the paper in the pool that is in your hands.)

LESSON EXTENSION IDEAS: Give the children a bag to save the paper they cut. As they leave the cutting pool, the children will take their bag of cut paper to a table to create a collage.

HOW TO CHECK FOR STUDENT UNDERSTANDING: As you monitor the children, keep a checklist to document their grip and fine motor cutting progress.

ACCOMMODATIONS FOR DIVERSE LEARNERS (SPECIAL NEEDS): You may want to get into the pool one-on-one with a child that needs direct instruction. If the pool is not accessible to a child, you can spread paper around a child either on a table or on the floor.

EVALUATION OF THE LESSON: The teacher will evaluate the activity using the checklists to determine the effectiveness of the activity. Through observation determine the enjoyment and interactions of the children.

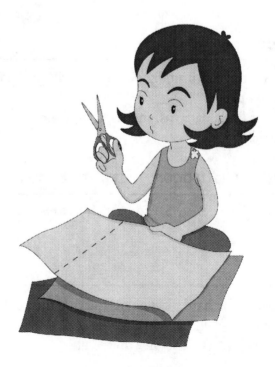

ACTIVITY 5

FRIENDS SCAVENGER HUNT

GOAL:

To promote an understanding and appreciation of diversity.

OBJECTIVE:

The children will complete a "Friend Scavenger Hunt" sheet to learn about the things that make each person in the classroom special.

Developmental Domain(s) Met:

Physical – Children will walk around the classroom and find classmates who help them complete the "Friends Scavenger Hunt" sheet.

Social/Emotional – Children will work together to find all the items on the "Friends Scavenger Hunt" sheet.

Language and Communication – Children will talk to the teacher and to each other about who meets the "Friends Scavenger Hunt" sheet items.

Cognitive – Children will understand that different classmates have different eye color; are left or right handed; have blond, red, or brown hair; have a brother or sister; have a dog or cat; or were born in a particular town.

Creative – Children will draw "self-portraits" showing what makes them special.

Materials Needed:

* Book: *We Share One World* by Jane Hoffelt
* "Friends Scavenger Hunt" sheet (teacher and children will decide what items to put on the list)

Environment (Indoor/Outdoor, Size of Group):

Classroom.

Procedure:

The teacher will read the book and introduce the idea of a "Friends Scavenger Hunt" during group time.

- Talk to the children about how our differences make us special.
- Guide the children to create a list of differences to include on the "Friends Scavenger Hunt" sheet.
- The children will take the sheet and find a friend who fits one of the differences listed.
- Children will have the friend write their name next to the item on the list that matches them.
- When the children have all completed the "Friends Scavenger Hunt" sheet, talk about what the experience was like for the children during group time.
- Help children understand that their differences make them special and make the entire class more special.

Questions for Children:

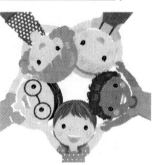

- Ask children, what does it mean to be different?
- What does it mean to be the same?
- Explain that everyone has differences and we are special because of our differences.

LESSON EXTENSION IDEAS:

- The book center will have books available on children from around the world. Books on children with special needs will also be available.
- A guest speaker may be invited to the classroom that day to talk about working with children who have special needs.
- The dramatic play area will have clothing from around the world.
- The music area will have folk songs from around the world

ACCOMMODATIONS FOR DIVERSE LEARNERS (SPECIAL NEEDS):
All children should be able to participate in this activity.

HOW TO CHECK FOR STUDENT UNDERSTANDING: Ask the children if they understand what it means to be the same or different. Then ask why it is a good to have differences in their classroom. What are some of the differences we have in this classroom?

EVALUATION OF THE LESSON: The teacher will evaluate the lesson based on the number of children who can complete the "Friends Scavenger Hunt" page and answer the diversity questions to show they appreciate differences.

ACTIVITY 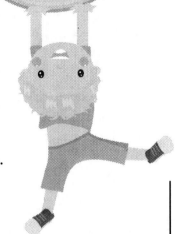 6

FUN WITH COMMUNITY HELPERS

GOAL:
To learn about community helpers and their roles.

OBJECTIVE:
The children will learn about community helpers and play a game related to community helpers.

Developmental Domain(s) Met:

Physical – The children will use motor skills to act out community helper roles.

Social/Emotional – The children will play a game with their peers.

Language and Communication – The children will communicate facts about community helpers.

Cognitive – The children will recall facts about community helpers.

Creative – The children will create a picture of a community helper.

Materials Needed:

* Book, *Whose Hat Is This?* by Sharon Katz Cooper, or any book about community helpers
* White construction paper
* Crayons or markers

Environment (Indoor/Outdoor, Size of Group):

Any size group in the classroom, seated on a rug.

Procedure:

The teacher will begin the lesson by reading the book, *Whose Hat Is This?* or any story about community helpers.

- Ask questions related to the book.
- Have children name as many community helpers as they can recall.
- Play charades with the children. A student will act out what a specific community helper does and the other children will try to guess which community helper it is. Suggestions: Police office, teacher, firefighter, nurse/doctor/dentist, baker, construction worker, mail carrier.
- Teach children the song about community helpers (see below).
- Have each child draw a picture of a community helper of their choice.

Community Helpers Song
(Tune: Mary had a Little Lamb)

The mailman helps deliver the mail, deliver the mail, deliver the mail. The mailman helps deliver the mail, that's what the mailman does.

The police man helps to keep us safe…..
The dentist helps to clean our teeth…….
The firefighter helps to put out the fire….
The teacher helps us learn and think….
The doctor keeps us healthy and strong….

The children can think of other community helpers and add verses to the song.

Questions for Children:

- What is a community?
- What is a community helper?
- How many community helpers can you name?
- How do community helpers help in the community?
- What do you want to do when you grow up?

LESSON EXTENSION IDEAS: Gather community helper props to place in the dramatic play area (firefighter's hat, construction worker's hat, police officer's hat and badge, doctor/nurse kit, mail carrier bag and envelopes). The children can act out various community helpers in the dramatic play area.

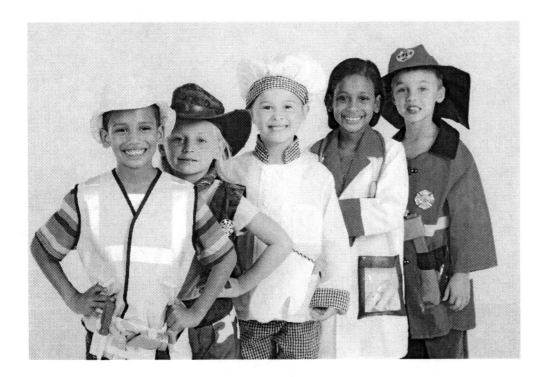

HOW TO CHECK FOR STUDENT UNDERSTANDING: The teacher will evaluate the students on their understanding of community helpers by taking notes on each child's response to the questions.

ACCOMMODATIONS FOR DIVERSE LEARNERS (SPECIAL NEEDS): Students with special needs may need help playing the charades game. They should be paired up with another student.

EVALUATION OF THE LESSON: The teacher will evaluate the lesson based on the participation, comprehension, and enjoyment of the children.

ACTIVITY 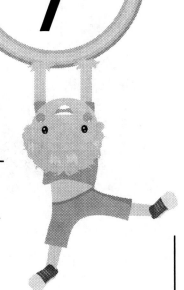 7

I CAN DO IT

GOAL:

To promote independence and build self-esteem.

OBJECTIVE:

The children will be able to complete an obstacle course.

Developmental Domain(s) Met:

Physical Health – The children will complete an obstacle course using their large and small motor skills.

Social/Emotional – The children will work together to make it through the obstacle course.

Language and Communication – The children will talk to the teacher and to each other about the obstacle course and the challenges they might face.

Cognitive – The teacher will encourage the children to use their critical thinking skills to figure out how to complete the obstacle course.

Creative – The teacher and students can help plan and create the obstacle course.

Materials Needed:

* Book: *We're Going on a Lion Hunt* by David Axtell
* Items for the obstacle course such as Hula Hoops, plastic cones, large blocks, playground items such as wagons, balance beam, sand box, glider, play tunnel

Environment (Indoor/Outdoor, Size of Group):

Indoors and outdoors, children will work as a group and in pairs.

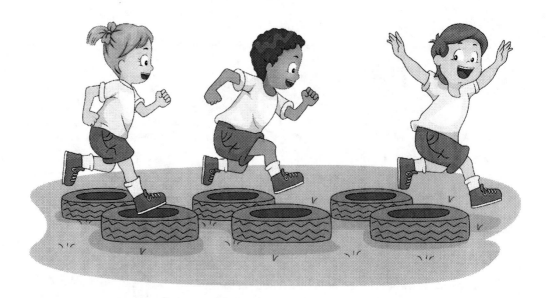

Procedure and Questions:

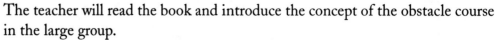

The teacher will read the book and introduce the concept of the obstacle course in the large group.

- Ask the children if they have ever completed an obstacle course.
- Has anyone had to overcome any challenges in their lives (tried to make a new friend, learn how to tie their shoes) and was it difficult?
- How were you able to do it successfully?
- Encourage the children to come up with items to put on the obstacle course and decide where they will get the items.
- Do you think you can make it through the obstacle course?
- How can you help your friends if they get stuck?
- Take the children outside and collectively decide where to put the items on the obstacle course.
- Direct the children to break into pairs and navigate the obstacle course.

LESSON EXTENSION IDEAS:

- Create a small obstacle course for inside the classroom so the children can rehearse before going outside.
- Children can create signs with directional markers for the obstacle course in the art center.
- Books on overcoming obstacles should be available in the reading center.

HOW TO CHECK FOR STUDENT UNDERSTANDING: Ask the children if they know what an obstacle course is and what it means to overcome a challenge. Then ask the children if they were able to help each other through the obstacle course. The teacher will ask the children how it made them feel when they got stuck and how they felt when they completed the challenge.

ACCOMMODATIONS FOR DIVERSE LEARNERS (SPECIAL NEEDS):

The teacher will determine the need for special accommodations for any children who have difficulty maneuvering through the course. The teacher will make sure the obstacle course is accessible.

EVALUATION OF THE LESSON:

The lesson would be evaluated four ways:

1. The number of children who were able to complete the obstacle course.
2. The number of children who were able to follow directions.
3. The number of children who were able to help others.
4. The number of children who understood the relationship between challenges in life and challenges in an obstacle course.

ACTIVITY 8

LET'S GO SHOPPING

GOAL:

To promote healthy food choices for preschool children.

OBJECTIVE:

The children will be introduced to how to create
a healthy shopping list from the main food groups.

Developmental Domain(s) Met:

- Physical – Children will help create a grocery store dramatic play area and a shopping list using their large and small motor skills.
- Social/Emotional – Children will work as a team to create the grocery store and shopping list with the teacher and the other children.
- Language and Communication – Children will discuss creating the grocery store and making the healthy choices grocery list with the teacher and the other children.
- Cognitive – Children will understand the concept of making a list and using it to go grocery shopping. They will go through the motions of shopping for healthy foods and making healthy snacks.
- Creative – Children will use the dramatic play center to dress like shoppers, grocery store clerks, and cooks.

Materials Needed:

- Book: *Maisy goes Shopping* by Lucy Cousins
- All types of grocery store items such as fruit, vegetables, dairy products and meat
- A table to set up a grocery store
- Reusable shopping bags
- Costumes from dramatic play area

* Grocery ads from the local supermarkets
* Poster materials, markers, paper, pencils, scissors, labels
* Toy cash register
* Monopoly money

Environment (Indoor/Outdoor, Size of Group):

Indoor/Outdoor

Procedure:

The teacher will read the book and introduce the lesson on healthy choices at the grocery store.

• Explain how important it is to eat the proper foods (fruits, vegetables, grains, and proteins). The teacher will talk about various types of healthy foods and how the children can keep their bodies healthy and strong by eating the right foods.

• Ask the children if they eat any special types of food at home. Some children can explain what it means to be vegetarian, vegan, or any other special diet choices.

• The teacher can also explain that some children have allergies to certain foods.

• Show pictures of the various food groups and help the children create a grocery list.

• Once the list is developed, the children will take on the various roles of the grocery store cashier, shoppers, and baggers.

• The children will act out the grocery shopping experience while they check off the healthy food item choices on their list.

• The children will then make a healthy snack using the items they purchased at the store.

Questions for the Children:

• What kinds of items did you put on the healthy choices grocery list?
• Why did you choose those items?
• Give examples of food items that are not healthy and ask the children why they are not healthy (candy, chips and soda).
• How can having a list help you and your family make good choices at the grocery store?

LESSON EXTENSION IDEAS: Plan a field trip to the local supermarket and take a tour of the various store departments. Allow children to ask the tour guide questions about healthy food choices at the store.

HOW TO CHECK FOR STUDENT UNDERSTANDING: The teacher will ask the children to give examples of healthy and not healthy food choices. The teacher will ask the children how they can keep their bodies healthy and what snacks are good for them.

ACCOMMODATIONS FOR DIVERSE LEARNERS (SPECIAL NEEDS): The grocery store must be accessible to all the children.

EVALUATION OF THE LESSON: The teacher will evaluate the lesson based on the number of children who can list healthy food choices and healthy snacks.

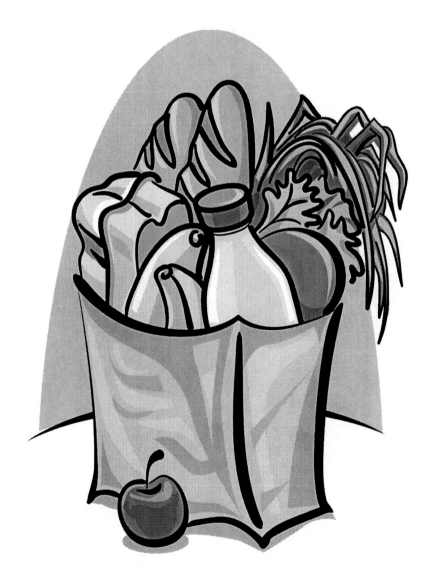

ACTIVITY 9

MY FAMILY AND ME

GOAL:

To appreciate their own family and the diversity of the other children and families in the class.

OBJECTIVE:

The children will be able to tell the class about their family by making a poster with the assistance and props from the teacher.

Developmental Domain(s) Met:

Physical – Children will use their fine motor skills to cut out pictures from magazines and glue items to a poster that depict various characteristics of their families.

Language and Communication – Children will talk to each other and to the teacher about families.

Cognitive – Children must understand that not every family is necessarily the same as theirs and that each family is special in it's own way.

Creative – Children will construct posters depicting what makes their family special.

Materials Needed:

* Book: *The Family Book* by Todd Parr
* Poster boards
* Glue
* Children's scissors
* Crayons
* Magazines
* Pictures of family members

Environment (Indoor/Outdoor, Size of Group):

Classroom, children will work individually.

Procedure and Questions:

The teacher will begin by reading the book and introduce the topic of families and explain that all families are not necessarily the same.

- Further explain that each family is special in it's own unique way.
- Note: Teacher will have previously told the children to bring in pictures of their family and magazines to be used to create their posters.
- Children will create "My Family and Me" posters. They may use pictures they brought in or cut pictures out of the magazines or both. They can also draw on the posters.
- After the children finish making their posters, they will share their family poster with the rest of the class.

ACCOMMODATIONS FOR DIVERSE LEARNERS (SPECIAL NEEDS):
All children should be included in this activity regardless of special needs.

LESSON EXTENSION IDEAS: Books on the topic of families should be available in the reading center.

HOW TO CHECK FOR STUDENT UNDERSTANDING:
The teacher will observe to see if each child understands how to make a poster of their family and understands that not all families are the same but they are all special in their own way.

EVALUATION OF THE
LESSON: Teachers can evaluate the lesson based on the number of children who can create a "My Family and Me" poster and share what makes their family special.

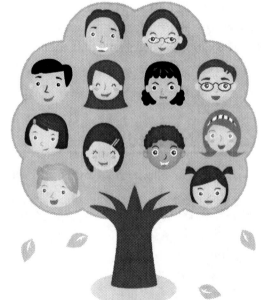

ACTIVITY 10

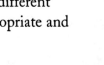

MY FEELINGS ARE OKAY

GOAL:

To let children know that feelings are normal reactions and to explain appropriate ways to react to those feelings.

OBJECTIVE:

The children will participate in a discussion of what causes different feelings and act out how to express emotions in both inappropriate and appropriate ways.

Developmental Domain(s) Met:

Social/Emotional – Expression of feelings.
Language and Communication – Discussion and verbal expression.
Creative – Acting.

Materials Needed:

 A book about feelings

Environment (Indoor/Outdoor, Size of Group):

Indoor or outdoor with space for acting out scenarios.

Procedure and Questions:

- Ask the children "what are feelings or emotions?" Discuss their responses.
- Read a children's book about feelings.
- Ask the children to make a sad, mad, excited, scared, and happy face. "What can make you feel these emotions? Why?"
- Ask the children, "who would like to stand up and act out their feelings?"

- Give these children a situation to act out with ground rules that allow no physical contact of aggression. Scenarios can include:
  - A friend says hi to you and gives you a big smile
  - Someone takes away your toy
  - You get to go on a trip
  - Someone hits you
  - There is a bad storm
  - You fall and hurt yourself
- Ask the children the right and wrong ways to act when these things happen. Compare the possible outcomes and guide them as needed toward appropriate ways to cope with feelings.

LESSON EXTENSION IDEAS:
- Four years and up - Give each child a plain sheet of white paper folded into four sections. In each corner of each section have them draw a small circle face:
  1. A happy face
  2. A sad face (upside down mouth, tears)
  3. A mad face (straight mouth, angled line for eyebrows)
  4. An excited face (big open smile).
- Ask them to draw something that makes them feel like the face they see in that section.

HOW TO CHECK FOR STUDENT UNDERSTANDING: Observe responses as you have the children express their emotions and act out scenarios.

ACCOMMODATIONS FOR DIVERSE LEARNERS (SPECIAL NEEDS): It may be necessary with some children to help them express themselves in a nurturing environment. Use books in a one-on-one setting to assist in helping children understand that emotions are normal and that they are free to express themselves appropriately without fear of consequences.

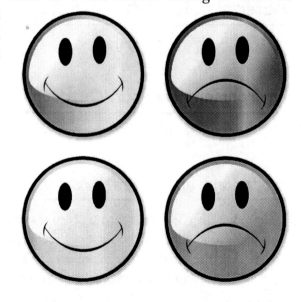

EVALUATION OF THE LESSON: The teacher will evaluate the activity based on subsequent observations of children's behavior and reactions to their feelings.

ACTIVITY 11

PLAY SAFE

GOAL:

To be able to play safely on the playground.

OBJECTIVE:

The children will be introduced to safe ways to
play on a playground and avoid hurting themselves or others.

Developmental Domain(s) Met: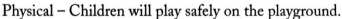

Physical – Children will play safely on the playground.

Social/Emotional – Children will learn to take care of themselves and
others when playing on the playground.

Language and Communication – Children will talk to each other and to
the teacher about playing safely on the playground.

Cognitive – Children must be able to understand that certain activities may
result in injuries to themselves or others while playing on the playground.

Creative – Children will develop a game to play on the playground that is
both fun and safe.

Materials Needed:

* Book: *Please Play Safe! Penguin's Guide To Playground Safety* by Margery
Cuyler
* A playground

Environment (Indoor/Outdoor, Size of Group):

Start in the classroom, then move to the playground.

Procedure and Questions:

The teacher will begin by reading the book and stressing the importance of playing safe on the playground. The teacher will then go over a list* of safe-play activities such as:

- There should always be a teacher or other adult present on the playground.
- Always pick up any trash on the playground to avoid getting cut.
- If a piece of playground equipment is broken, don't play on it, alert a teacher.
- Be safe on the swings; always sit on the swing, slow down before you get off a swing, and don't walk or play to close to someone who is swinging, you could get hit.
- Always use both hands when you climb.
- Never climb up the front of the slide.
- Always slide feet first.
- Only one person can slide at a time.

*Note: The teacher may have to modify this list based on their particular playground.

- Take the children to the playground and have them practice safe-play activities following the teacher's directions.
- Next the children will create their own safe and fun playground game.

ACCOMMODATIONS FOR DIVERSE LEARNERS (SPECIAL NEEDS):
All children should be included in this activity regardless of special needs.

HOW TO CHECK FOR STUDENT UNDERSTANDING: The teacher will evaluate whether or not the game the children create follows the safe-play guidelines.

EVALUATION OF THE LESSON: Teachers can evaluate the lesson based on the number of children who can remember the guidelines and play safe on the playground.

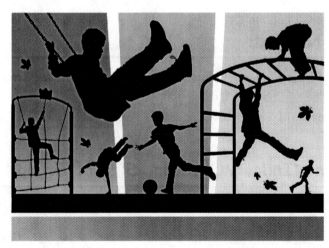

ACTIVITY 12

RESCUE ME

GOAL:
To teach children not to be afraid but to be aware of their surroundings.

OBJECTIVE:
The children will learn what to do if they are afraid, who to ask for help, and how to call 911.

Developmental Domain(s) Met:

Physical – Children will use their fine motor skills to create a poster and learn to call 911 on a phone.

Social/Emotional – Children will learn to understand what it means to be afraid and how to ask for help.

Language and Communication – Children will talk to each other and to the teacher about what it means to be afraid, who to ask for help, and how and when to call 911.

Cognitive – Children must understand that you only call 911 in an emergency and that there are certain people in the community you can ask to help you if you are afraid.

Creative – Children will create a poster with pictures of the people they can go to if they ever need help. They will also glue a picture of a phone on the poster and draw the numbers 911.

Materials Needed:

* Book: *It's Time to Call 911: What to do in an Emergency* by Inc. Penton Overseas
* Posters
* Pictures of police, firefighters, medical professionals, teachers, and parents
* Picture of a phone to cut out and glue on the poster

* Cut-out numbers 9-1-1
* Glue
* Children's scissors
* Crayons

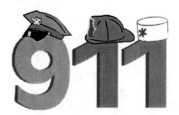

Environment (Indoor/Outdoor, Size of Group):

Classroom, children will work individually.

Procedure and Questions:

- The teacher will begin by reading the book.
- Introduce the topic of what to do if you are afraid, who to ask for help, and how to call 911 in an emergency.
- Explain that there are lots of reasons you might be afraid but you do not always call 911.
- Have you ever been afraid?
- Explain that when they are afraid, it is good to get away from the situation and find people they can ask for help.
- Talk about going places in pairs and how it helps people to be less afraid if they are with someone else.
- Explain that you only call 911 when someone is hurt.
- If you are afraid for other reasons; you talk to a parent, teacher, policeman, firefighter, or someone else you know will help you.
- Have the children make a poster with pictures of the people they can go to for help.
- Have the children cut out a picture of a phone and glue it on the poster.
- The children will write the numbers 9-1-1 on the poster.

ACCOMMODATIONS FOR DIVERSE LEARNERS (SPECIAL NEEDS):
All children should be included in this activity regardless of special needs.

LESSON EXTENSION IDEAS: Books on the topic of community helpers should be available in the reading center.

HOW TO CHECK FOR STUDENT UNDERSTANDING: The teacher will have each child create a poster with the people in their lives they can go to if they are afraid. The teacher will have the children glue a phone and the numbers 911 on their posters. The teacher will ask the children what they should do if they are afraid and when they should call 911.

EVALUATION OF THE LESSON: Teachers can evaluate the lesson based on the number of children who can explain what to do if they are afraid, who to ask for help, and when to call 911.

ACTIVITY 13

THIS IS MY HOME

GOAL:

The children will describe their home environment and the relationship to the community.

OBJECTIVE:

The children will create a simple house and dictate information about their home and community.

Developmental Domain(s) Met:

Physical – Fine motor: cutting, gluing, and drawing.
Social/Emotional – Expressing familiarity and belonging as well as a sense of community and cooperative art.
Language and Communication – Dictation.
Creative – Artistic representation.

Materials Needed:

* A book about different types of homes
* One 9 x 12 piece of construction paper per child (You may want to prepare the paper beforehand by having a volunteer lightly draw dashed lines where the paper is to be folded and solid lines where the paper is to be cut as explained below under Procedure.)
* One roll of butcher paper or newsprint paper
* Children's scissors
* Oil pastels, markers, or crayons
* Glue

Environment (Indoor/Outdoor, Size of Group):

Indoor or outdoor. Group size 8 to 12 (this activity is best with 4-year-olds and older).

Procedure and Questions

- Read book to children.
- Ask the children about their home.
  - What do they like about it?
  - What color is it?
  - Who lives in their home?
  - Do they have pets?
  - What do they walk or drive by on their way to school?
- Model how to fold and cut the paper to turn it into a house.
- Holding the paper vertically, fold down each top corner forming a point (rooftop). At the bottom of the paper below the rooftop, cut a door flap.
- Model how to draw squares and circles to represent windows.
- Glue down on long sheet of butcher paper.
- As children work on their houses, write down their responses to the questions.
- The children will create a group mural. Have them glue down their houses on the butcher paper and draw roads, trees, flowers, pets, and people between the houses.
- If they children can, have them write their name by their house.
- Type what they told you and glue down next to their home.

LESSON EXTENSION IDEAS:
- Discuss local community helpers and local businesses.
- Bring in environmental print of words and logos the children will recognize.
- Have the children add cut-out buildings representing local businesses.

HOW TO CHECK FOR STUDENT UNDERSTANDING: Observe and record the ability of the children to describe their home environment.

ACCOMMODATIONS FOR DIVERSE LEARNERS (SPECIAL NEEDS):
Assist children with fine motor difficulties that are unable to fold, cut, and/or draw. Introduce descriptive words and show examples of those words.

EVALUATION OF THE LESSON: The teacher will evaluate the lesson based on the children's ability to verbalize characteristics of their home and community as well as their ability to work with others to create a community mural.

ACTIVITY 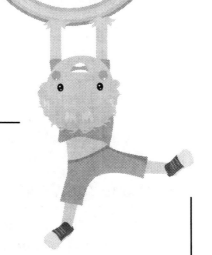 14

WAVING STREAMERS

GOAL:

To enjoy music and movement.

OBJECTIVE:

The children will be able to move to music in creative ways.

Developmental Domain(s) Met:

Physical – The children will use fine and gross motor skills while waving crepe paper to music.

Social/Emotional – The children will cooperate with each other in a movement activity.

Creative – The children will move in creative ways while waving crepe paper streamers.

Materials Needed:

* Brightly colored crepe paper cut in 2-foot strips, holiday colors such as red and green for Christmas can be used
* CD player and CD, or other form of music player

Environment (Indoor/Outdoor, Size of Group):

Small group in the classroom standing apart from each other.

Procedure:

• Pass out a long strip of crepe paper to each child.

- Demonstrate how to wave the crepe paper to music, such as fast and slow, above the head, in circular motions, up and down.
- Play a selection of music and the children will move and wave their streamers. "Dance of the Sugar Plum Fairy" by Tchaikovsky works well for this activity.

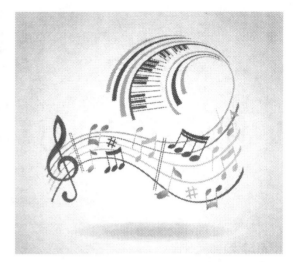

Questions for Children:

- What color is your streamer?
- How many [color of streamer] streamers do you see?
- Can we make a pattern with the streamers?
- Can you wave your streamer fast? Slow?

LESSON EXTENSION IDEAS: The children will wave the streamers to an upbeat, fast song. Have children glue their streamers on a class mural after the movement activity is completed.

HOW TO CHECK FOR STUDENT UNDERSTANDING: The teacher will check for understanding by noting which students were able to use their motor skills to manipulate the streamer.

ACCOMMODATIONS FOR DIVERSE LEARNERS (SPECIAL NEEDS): Students with special needs will stand near the teacher for additional assistance when needed.

EVALUATION OF THE LESSON: The teacher will evaluate the students based on their participation and enjoyment.

ACTIVITY 15

WHO'S IN A FAMILY?

GOAL:

To help children be aware that family is made up of people who love and support you.

OBJECTIVE:

The children will bring photos or draw pictures of people who are important to them and share them with others.

Developmental Domain(s) Met:

Physical – Fine motor: drawing.
Social/Emotional – Relationships.
Language and Communication – Sharing time.
Cognitive – Matching.

Materials Needed:

* A book about families (conventional and non-conventional)
* Pictures or posters of families
* Photos that the children brought in of their families
* Drawing paper (for those who do not bring in photos)

Environment (Indoor/Outdoor, Size of Group):

Indoor, group size 8 to 12.

Procedure and Questions:

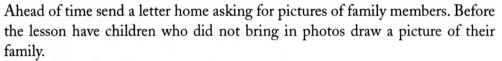

Ahead of time send a letter home asking for pictures of family members. Before the lesson have children who did not bring in photos draw a picture of their family.

- Read a book about families of all kinds.
- Reflect on the book allowing the children to ask questions.
- Have children sit in a circle on the floor.
- Put all of the children's photos and drawings in a basket in the middle of the circle.
- Ask open-ended questions of the children.

> Who is in your family?
> Who do you love?
> Why are these people important to you?
> Are all families the same?

One at a time, let the children pull a random picture or drawing out of the basket and guess who it belongs to. Whoever the picture belongs to gets to tell everyone about their family and then draw the next one out of the basket. Continue until all children have had a turn.

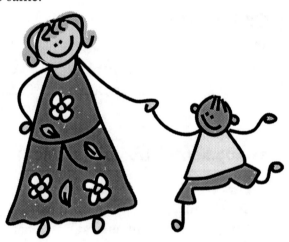

LESSON EXTENSION IDEAS:

- Create a family book that the children can check out to take home.
- Set up a play house and figures in a center. Be sure to have a diverse group of people figures.

HOW TO CHECK FOR STUDENT UNDERSTANDING: Record responses to the open ended questions.

ACCOMMODATIONS FOR DIVERSE LEARNERS (SPECIAL NEEDS): For children that have difficulty speaking in front of others, have them sit with you and ask them questions about their picture.

EVALUATION OF THE LESSON: The teacher will evaluate the activity based on the social and emotional involvement of the children and their interest in describing their family.

ACTIVITY 16

WIGGLES AND WAGGLES

GOAL:

To understand the importance of exercise in the daily routine.

OBJECTIVE:

The children will participate in spontaneous directed exercise throughout the day.

Developmental Domain(s) Met:

Physical – Children will follow teacher's directions throughout the day and use their large and small motor skills to perform physical activities.

Social/Emotional – Children will recognize that they feel happier and have more fun with their friends when they are physically active.

Language and Communication – Children will talk to each other and to the teacher about the movements and exercise they are doing.

Cognitive – Children will listen and follow directions.

Creative – Children will be spontaneous and create movements to the music provided by the teacher.

Materials Needed:

 Book: *Spriggles Motivational Books for Children: Activity & Exercise* by Jeff Gottlieb and Martha Gottlieb

 Any device able to play music (CD, DVD, computer)

Environment (Indoor/Outdoor, Size of Group):

Classroom, children will work individually.

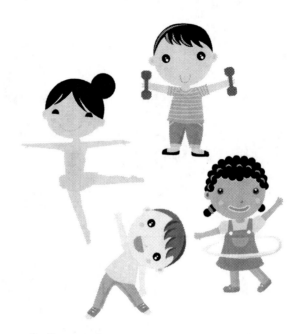

Procedure and Questions:

The teacher will begin by reading the book and talk to the children about how important it is to exercise everyday.

- Talk about eating healthy food, getting lots of sleep and exercising to stay healthy.
- Explain that healthy minds and bodies need exercise everyday.
- Turn on the music throughout the day and the children can be as creative as they want. For example, when music is played, the children can create their own dance, hop, skip, or jump to it.
- Explain that the children must not touch any other student while they are doing their exercise.
- Did you like exercising to the music?
- Why is exercise important?
- Put the music on again and allow the children to create their own exercise.

ACCOMMODATIONS FOR DIVERSE LEARNERS (SPECIAL NEEDS):
All children should be included in this activity regardless of special needs.

LESSON EXTENSION IDEAS: Books on the topic of exercise should be available in the reading center.

HOW TO CHECK FOR STUDENT UNDERSTANDING: The teacher will have each child create a simple exercise and ask them why exercise is important.

EVALUATION OF THE LESSON: Teachers can evaluate the lesson based on the number of children who can follow her directions, create their own exercise to music, and explain why exercise is important.

ACTIVITY 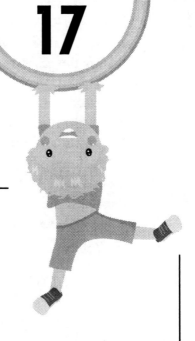 17

IT'S MY TURN!

GOAL:

To promote positive relationships in the group.

OBJECTIVE:

Create steps for improving group relationships
during center group times.

Developmental Domain(s) Met:

Physical – Students will be aware of the conflict between two or more
students and make sure they are not involved.

Social/Emotional – Students who are involved in the conflict will learn
ways to work through each situation with a conflict resolution plan given
by the teacher.

Language and Communication – Students will learn to verbally express
themselves with words not actions.

Cognitive – Students will learn the steps of conflict resolution in order to
facilitate group activity as a positive.

Creative – With the teacher's help or a visiting counselor students will
create nonverbal signs to use when a possible conflict begins.

Environment (Indoor/Outdoor, Size of Group):

Classroom

Procedure and Questions:

The teacher will introduce the concept of conflict resolution to the group as a
response to an incident that happen during small group center time. She will

explain the steps in helping to solve the conflict and how each child can learn to benefit from these strategies:

1. Cool down – take a step back, deep breath, and relax. What just happened and why? Let's talk about it.
2. Identify the problem – make sure you find out what the real problem is, let each child express their version, make sure there are no interruptions by the other child when one is talking.
3. What's the real problem here? What are you really worried about?
4. Brainstorm a solution – Get input from each child involved and then talk about possible workable solutions
5. Try one out – Let's see if one of our ideas works? If not, then what are next steps?
6. Follow-up - Let's make sure we don't have this problem again. How can we do that?

PRESENT THE SITUATION AS IT OCCURRED:

Sample

Computer time center: Johnny and Sylvia have both been assigned computer time – one AFTER the other. Sylvia has decided she wants to go first BEFORE Johnny. Abraham is already on the computer and is not finished with his project. He doesn't want to leave even though his time his up.

Sylvia announces to Abraham that his time is up. Johnny says, "No, it's my time – look at my name on the sign up chart". Abraham says, "I'm NOT getting up" so both Johnny and Sylvia attempt to push Abraham off the chair. At this time the teacher realizes what is happening and takes all 3 children to a quiet corner for a conversation.

STEPS FOR CHILDREN INPUT: What happens next? How would you handle this problem?

HOW TO CHECK FOR STUDENT UNDERSTANDING: How would you check for whether or not the children understand what happened and whether their solutions to solve the problem would work?

ACCOMMODATIONS FOR DIVERSE LEARNERS: Special needs children would need individual guidance to make sure all directions were understood.

EVALUATION OF THE LESSON: Depending on the solutions given by the children, either individually or as a group, you could see if the conflict resolution steps were followed. If not, what would the next steps be in the process?

Section 4

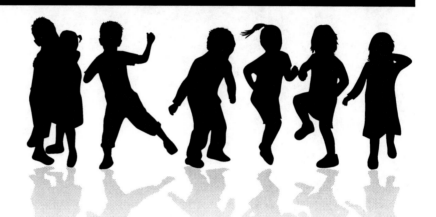

FINE ARTS

Fine arts play an important role in the development and learning experiences of young children. Children are naturally interested in drawing, dancing, singing, poetry, and expressing themselves. Teachers who incorporate the fine arts into the curriculum, give young children opportunities to express themselves and develop a sense of self-worth. Studies indicate that a program rich in the arts leads to higher achievement in other academic areas.

The fine arts section of this book includes activities that encourage creativity and imagination in young children. The activities are hands-on and easy to use for teachers with or without musical abilities. The materials are easily accessible and economical. The children are encouraged to use their imagination and creativity while enjoying the arts!

ACTIVITY 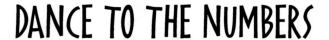 1

DANCE TO THE NUMBERS

GOAL:

To combine creative movement with basic math concepts.

OBJECTIVE:

The children will follow simple directions to create a
dance involving body movement and numbers.

Developmental Domain(s) Met:

Physical – Children will follow teacher's directions to move forward, back,
side-to-side, and hopping and clapping.

Language and Communication – Children will talk to each other and to the
teacher about the dance they are creating.

Cognitive – Children must be able to count from one to five and be able to
recognize patterns.

Materials Needed:

* Book: *Giraffe's Can't Dance* by Giles Andreae
* Any device able to play music (CD, DVD, computer)

Environment (Indoor/Outdoor, Size of Group):

Classroom, children will work as a group.

Procedure and Questions:

The teacher will begin by reading the book and ensure children can count from
one to five.

* Explain that a dance is really a series of patterns.

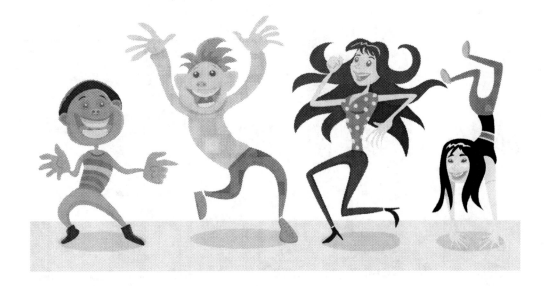

- Demonstrate by moving forward and back or side-to-side while clapping and counting from one to five (make up any dance pattern).
- Teach the children to follow the steps—be as creative as you want. For example, take three steps forward, then three steps back; then one step to the right and two steps to the left. Clap your hands over your head five times. This is an example of a simple dance pattern.
- Did you like dancing to the numbers?
- Why is dancing a pattern? (A dance is learning a series of patterns.)
- Reflect on the book you read with the children and ask if everyone can dance.
- Explain that everyone can dance in some form and not everyone's dance has to be the same.
- Put the music on again and allow the children to make up their own dance.

ACCOMMODATIONS FOR DIVERSE LEARNERS (SPECIAL NEEDS):
All children should be included in this activity regardless of special needs.

LESSON EXTENSION IDEAS: Books on the topic of dance movement or patterns should be available in the reading center.

HOW TO CHECK FOR STUDENT UNDERSTANDING: The teacher will have each child create a simple dance using the numbers one to five.

EVALUATION OF THE LESSON: Teachers can evaluate the lesson based on the number of children who can follow directions and dance to the numbers.

ACTIVITY 2

GUESS THE INSTRUMENT

GOAL:

To experience and enjoy music.

OBJECTIVE:

The children will be able to identify various rhythm instruments and recognize the sound the instrument makes.

Developmental Domain(s) Met:

Physical – The children will use fine motor skills when playing the instruments.

Social/Emotional – The children will learn to take turns playing instruments.

Language and Communication – The children will be able to identify instruments and describe what sound they make.

Creative – The children will express individual creativity when playing rhythm instruments.

Materials Needed:

* Various rhythm instruments such as tambourines, finger cymbals, triangles, jingle bells, and drums
* A puppet theater screen or some type of shield to hide behind when playing the instruments.

Environment (Indoor/Outdoor, Size of Group):

Small group seated on the floor in the classroom.

Procedure:

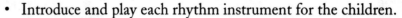

- Introduce and play each rhythm instrument for the children.
- Pass each instrument around the circle and let each child play the instruments.
- Hide behind a screen and play an instrument.
- The children will identify which instrument is being played.
- Give each child a turn to hide behind the screen and choose an instrument to play for the class. Two students may play at the same time.

Questions for the Children:

- What are the instruments?
- How do you play these instruments?
- What does the instrument sound like?

LESSON EXTENSION IDEAS: The children will be given the opportunity to play the instruments on their own. Other instruments could be added and played by the children.

HOW TO CHECK FOR STUDENT UNDERSTANDING: The children will be evaluated by teacher observation. The teacher will take notes on each child's participation and attention during the lesson.

ACCOMMODATIONS FOR DIVERSE LEARNERS (SPECIAL NEEDS): Students with special needs should be seated close to the teacher and be given assistance when playing instruments.

EVALUATION OF THE LESSON: The teacher will evaluate the lesson based on the children's enjoyment, participation, and comprehension.

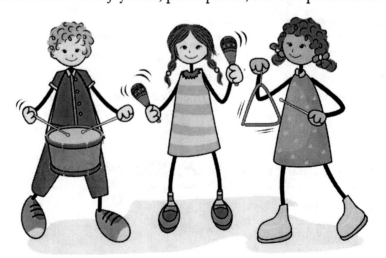

ACTIVITY 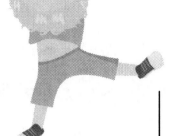 3

HOKEY POKEY VARIATIONS

GOAL:

To enjoy and experience music.

OBJECTIVE:

The children will be able to sing the Hokey Pokey and do the appropriate actions to the song.

Developmental Domain(s) Met:

Physical – The children will use motor skills when dancing to the Hokey Pokey.

Social/Emotional – The children will sing together as a group.

Language and Communication – The children will communicate words related to the theme that is being studied.

Cognitive – The children will remember the words to the song.

Creative – The children will think of new words to use in the song.

Materials Needed:

* A large area for the children to stand with their own space
* Music player with the song Hokey Pokey (CD, DVD, computer)

Environment (Indoor/Outdoor, Size of Group):

Indoor or outdoor, any size group.

Procedure:

The teacher will begin the lesson by singing or playing a CD with the song "The Hokey Pokey" on it.
- Demonstrate the actions for the song for the children.
- Encourage the children to try the actions.
- After the song ends, ask the children to change the words to the song by pretending to be an animal while singing the Hokey Pokey. Suggestions:

Squirrel for Fall

You put your bushy tail in, you put your bushy tail out, you put your bushy tail in and you shake it all about. You do the squirrel pokey and you turn yourself around. That's what it's all about!

Continue with: squirrel nose, squirrel paws, whole squirrel, squirrel cheeks. Ask the children what other parts of the squirrel they could use for the song.

Reindeer for Winter

You put your antlers in, you put your antlers out, you put your antlers in and you shake them all about. You do the reindeer pokey and you gallop yourself around. That's what it's all about!
Continue with: red nose, hoofs, reindeer tail.

Bunny for Spring
You put your bunny paws in, you put your bunny paws out, you put your bunny paws in and you shake them all about. You do the bunny pokey and you hop yourself around. That's what it's all about!
Continue with: bunny ears, bunny tail, bunny nose.

Questions for Children:

- What animal could we pretend to be while doing the Hokey Pokey?
- How many animal parts did we use in the song?
- If you could have any pet you wanted, what would that be?

LESSON EXTENSION IDEAS: The children could draw a picture of the animal acted out in the song or a pet they would like to have.

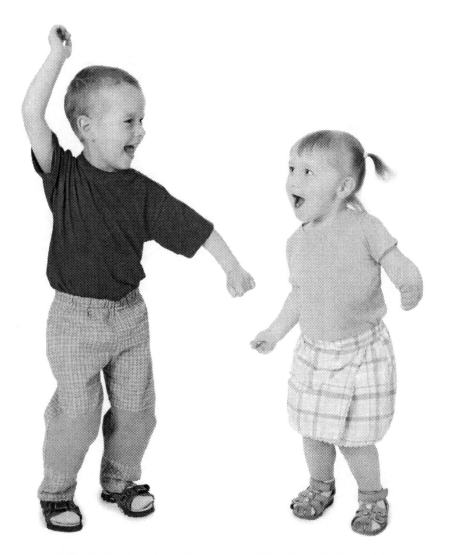

HOW TO CHECK FOR STUDENT UNDERSTANDING: The teacher will evaluate the students based on their participation and memory skills.

ACCOMMODATIONS FOR DIVERSE LEARNERS (SPECIAL NEEDS): Students with special needs should be placed close to the teacher.

EVALUATION OF THE LESSON: The teacher will evaluate the lesson based on the participation and enjoyment of the children.

ACTIVITY 4

JINGLE BELL BRACELETS

GOAL:
To enjoy music and shake instruments to the rhythm of a song.

OBJECTIVE:
The children will make a jingle bell bracelet and shake it to the rhythm of a song.

Developmental Domain(s) Met:

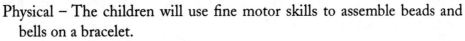

Physical – The children will use fine motor skills to assemble beads and bells on a bracelet.

Cognitive – The child will be able to count beads and bells, and identify colors of beads.

Creative – The children will use creativity when choosing colors and patterns for bracelet.

Materials Needed:

* Pipe cleaners
* Small colored beads
* Small bells that can be strung on a pipe cleaner

Environment (Indoor/Outdoor, Size of Group):

Small group in the classroom seated at tables.

Procedure:

The teacher will begin the lesson by shaking a jingle bell bracelet.

- Tell the children they are going to make their own bracelet out of beads and bells.
- Demonstrate how to make patterns with beads and bells.
- Seat children at the tables and allow them to assemble their beads and bells on a pipe cleaner.
- The teacher will twist the ends of the pipe cleaner making sure to tuck in the ends so that the wire doesn't scratch the children.

Questions for Children:

- What does the sound of the bells remind you of?
- How do you think you could make this bracelet?
- Do you know what a pattern is?
- Can you count the beads and bells?

LESSON EXTENSION IDEAS: The children could make patterns using various toys and objects in the classroom.

HOW TO CHECK FOR STUDENT UNDERSTANDING: The teacher will evaluate the lesson by noting which children were able to count, sort, and make patterns with the beads and bells.

ACCOMMODATIONS FOR DIVERSE LEARNERS (SPECIAL NEEDS): Students with special needs will need assistance from the teacher to make patterns and string the beads.

EVALUATION OF THE LESSON: The lesson will be evaluated and modified based on the teacher's observation of participation and enjoyment from the children.

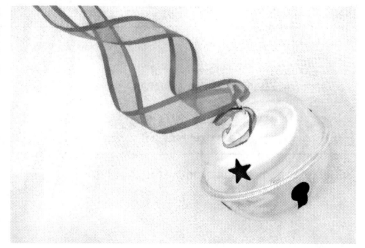

ACTIVITY 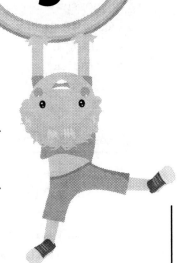 5

LOUD OR SOFT

GOAL:
To listen to music and determine if it is loud or soft.

OBJECTIVE:
The children will be able to listen to various selections of music and determine if the music is loud or soft.

Developmental Domain(s) Met:

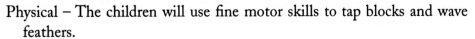

Physical – The children will use fine motor skills to tap blocks and wave feathers.

Social/Emotional – The children will interact with other children and the teacher.

Language and Communication – The children will be able to use language skills to communicate what he/she hears.

Materials Needed:

* Music CD and player with loud and soft music (classical music is good to use with this activity)
* Two small blocks for each child
* One large feather for each child

Environment (Indoor/Outdoor, Size of Group):

Small group in the classroom seated on the floor.

Procedure:

The teacher will begin the lesson with the children seated on the floor in a circle.
- Demonstrate how to tap the blocks together when loud music is played.
- Demonstrate how to blow on the feather or toss the feather in the air when soft music is played.
- Play the music for a while, allowing children to determine which action to perform.

Questions for Children:

- What do you think of when you hear the word soft?
- What do you think of when you hear the word loud?
- How many loud songs did you hear?
- How many soft songs did you hear?
- What does soft music remind you of?
- What does loud music remind you of?

LESSON EXTENSION IDEAS: The children can dance or march around the room while listening to loud/soft music.

HOW TO CHECK FOR STUDENT UNDERSTANDING: The teacher will keep a record of which children participated and understood the concept of loud and soft music.

ACCOMMODATIONS FOR DIVERSE LEARNERS (SPECIAL NEEDS): Children with special needs may need assistance from the teacher when manipulating blocks and feathers, or they could be paired with another child.

EVALUATION OF THE LESSON: The teacher will evaluate the lesson based on the children's participation and enjoyment.

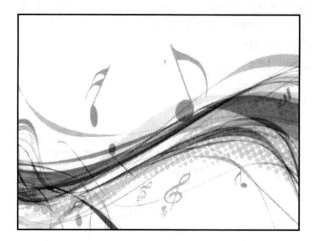

ACTIVITY 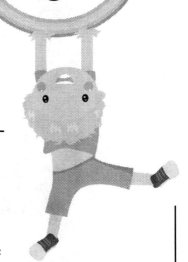 6

MARCHING BAND

> ### GOAL:
> To experience and enjoy music.
>
> ### OBJECTIVE:
> The children will play musical instruments while marching around in a circle.

Developmental Domain(s) Met:

Physical – The children will use motor skills to march and play instruments.

Social/Emotional – The children will interact with their peers while marching.

Creative – The children will express creativity when playing instruments.

Materials Needed:

* A variety of rhythm instruments: tambourines, shakers, bells, drums, triangles
* Marching music and player, American songs work well for this activity

Environment (Indoor/Outdoor, Size of Group):

Inside or outside, any size group.

Procedure:

The teacher will begin the lesson by demonstrating how to play each of the rhythm instruments.

- Allow children to come to the front of the class, one at a time and choose an instrument to play.

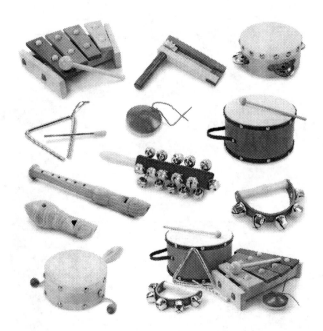

- The children will march around in a circle while playing their instruments. This activity works well outside also, as the children march in parade formation and play the instruments.
- Play a CD with marching music as the children play the instruments. American songs work well for this activity or any music that is lively and has a steady beat.

Questions for the Children:

- How many instruments can you see on the table?
- What do the instruments sound like?
- Can you clap to the beat of the music?

LESSON EXTENSION IDEAS: The children could exchange instruments and try to make up a song while playing the instrument.

HOW TO CHECK FOR STUDENT UNDERSTANDING: The teacher will take notes while observing the children to see if they are able to play the instruments correctly.

ACCOMMODATIONS FOR DIVERSE LEARNERS (SPECIAL NEEDS): Students with special needs may need assistance when playing the instruments.

EVALUATION OF THE LESSON: The teacher will evaluate the lesson based on whether or not the children are able to play the instruments and march at the same time.

ACTIVITY 7

MARSHMALLOW PAINTING

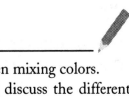

GOAL:

To learn about visual arts and color mixing.

OBJECTIVE:

The children will be able to identify what colors are produced when primary colors are mixed together.

Developmental Domain(s) Met:

Physical – The children will use fine motor skills when mixing colors.

Language and Communication – The children will discuss the different colors that are produced when mixing primary colors

Creative – The children will create a variety of colors by mixing them together.

Materials Needed:

* Book: *White Rabbit's Color Book* by Alan Baker
* Two paper plates per child
* Two tubes each of yellow, blue, and red gel frosting (this is enough for 12 students)
* One large marshmallow per child

Environment (Indoor/Outdoor, Size of Group):

In the classroom, sitting at tables.

Procedure:

The teacher will begin the lesson by reading the book, *White Rabbit's Color Book*.
- Demonstrate how to use a large marshmallow to mix the colors of frosting. (Use the marshmallow as a paint brush.)
- Use one plate for mixing, the other to paint on.

Questions for the Children:

- What happened to White Rabbit in the story?
- What are the three primary colors?
- What will happen if we mix the colors together?

LESSON EXTENSION IDEAS: Have children use <u>paint</u> to create a picture of their faces. Help them mix paint (pink, peach, white, and brown) to match the color of their skin.

HOW TO CHECK FOR STUDENT UNDERSTANDING: The children will be evaluated by teacher observation and taking note of which children participated and enjoyed the lesson.

ACCOMMODATIONS FOR DIVERSE LEARNERS (SPECIAL NEEDS): This lesson is beneficial to all students. Children with special needs may need assistance from the teacher or peers.

EVALUATION OF THE LESSON: The teacher will evaluate the lesson based on the enjoyment and creativity expressed by the children.

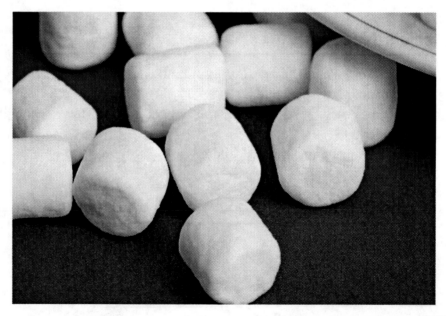

A C T I V I T Y   8

MUSICAL WATER GLASSES

GOAL:

To experience and enjoy music.

OBJECTIVE:

The children will be able to determine if water in glass containers makes a high or low pitch according to how much water is in the glass.

Developmental Domain(s) Met:

Physical – The children will use fine motor skills when tapping the glasses of water.

Language and Communication – The children will discuss with peers and teachers what they hear when tapping the glasses of water.

Creative – The children will be allowed to mix the colored water (with teacher assistance) to create new colors.

Materials Needed:

* Three large water glasses
* Food coloring
* A spoon or object for tapping the glasses
* Water

Environment (Indoor/Outdoor, Size of Group):

Classroom, small group of children is recommended.

Procedure:

- Show the children the water glasses filled with different levels of colored water. (You may add the food coloring in front of them if desired.)
- Experiment with different levels of water.
- Let each child have a turn tapping the glasses.

Questions for Children:

- What do you think will happen when these glasses are tapped with a spoon?
- Which glass of water makes a high sound?
- Which glass of water makes a low sound?
- If a glass is empty, what sound do you think it will make?
- What will happen if we mix the colors of water?

LESSON EXTENSION IDEAS: Children can draw a picture of each of the water glasses and dictate what happened when each glass was tapped. Children can play various rhythm instruments (triangle, cymbal, drum) and compare the sound they make to the sound made by the water glasses.

HOW TO CHECK FOR STUDENT UNDERSTANDING: The children will be evaluated by the teacher. Each child will be asked about the sound produced by the water glasses. The teacher will determine if the child understands how different levels of water produce different pitches. The teacher will keep a record of what each child said about the experiment.

ACCOMMODATIONS FOR DIVERSE LEARNERS (SPECIAL NEEDS): All children will benefit from this lesson. For a child with special needs, it is recommended that he/she is in the front of the classroom. For a child that is gifted, it is recommended that he/she explore the various pitches produced by the water on their own.

EVALUATION OF THE LESSON:
The teacher will evaluate the lesson by determining if each child understood the experiment and enjoyed the activity.

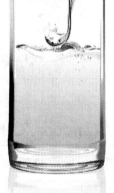
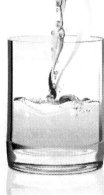

ACTIVITY 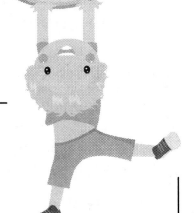 9

PASS THE HEART

GOAL:
To share feelings and thoughts.

OBJECTIVE:
The children will be able to express feelings after listening to music.

Developmental Domain(s) Met:

Physical – The children will use motor skills while playing a game.

Social/Emotional – The children will learn to express their feelings and thoughts.

Language and Communication – The children will be able to use words that express feelings and thoughts.

Creative – The children will think of words to express feelings and make a decorative heart picture.

Materials Needed:

* A stuffed heart or cardboard cut-out of a heart
* Soft, soothing music and a music player

Environment (Indoor/Outdoor, Size of Group):

Small group in the classroom seated on the floor.

Procedure:

• Begin the lesson by talking about feelings.

- Ask the children what words express feelings (happy, sad, angry, joyful, tired).
- Play soft music on a CD player as the children pass a stuffed heart (or heart shape) around the circle.
- When the music stops, the child holding the heart will say something nice about a friend or family member.
- Continue passing the heart until each child has had a turn.

Questions for Children:

- What are feelings?
- How do you feel today?
- What is something nice that you can say to someone?
- What are words that express feelings?

LESSON EXTENSION IDEAS: The children will go to the tables and decorate a heart cut-out with crayons, sequins, glitter, etc.

HOW TO CHECK FOR STUDENT UNDERSTANDING: The teacher will evaluate the children by writing down what each child says about their feelings.

ACCOMMODATIONS FOR DIVERSE LEARNERS (SPECIAL NEEDS): Children with special needs should receive guidance to help think of words to express feelings. They should be seated close to the teacher for assistance when needed.

EVALUATION OF THE LESSON: The teacher will evaluate the lesson based on the children's ability to express their feelings and their ability to say kind words to each other.

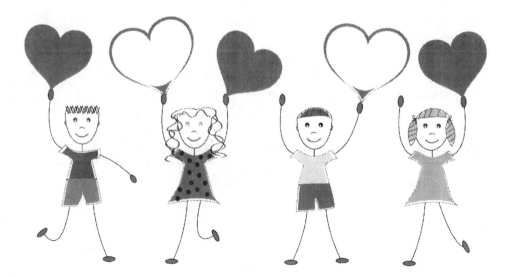

ACTIVITY 10

SHAKIN' EGGS!

GOAL:

To experience and enjoy music.

OBJECTIVE:

The children will be introduced to the concept
that music has a beat. The children will play instruments to the beat of
a song.

Developmental Domain(s) Met:

Physical – Children will shake eggs filled with Skittles or M&Ms.
Cognitive – Children will count the number of candies inside the egg.
Creative – Children will dance and move to the music in creative ways.

Materials Needed:

* One plastic egg for each child
* One large bag of
  Skittles or M&Ms
* Tape for sealing eggs
* Basket for eggs
* CD of lively music
  and music player
  (Raffi's CD "Baby

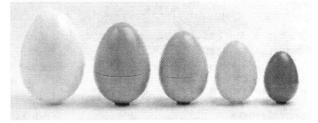

  Beluga" with the song "Day-Oh" works well for this lesson)

Environment (Indoor/Outdoor, Size of Group):

Classroom on a large rug is recommended. Up to 20 students.

Procedure:

Before the lesson, the teacher will prepare one plastic egg for each child by filling it with about 12-14 candies. (Either have two colors of eggs or two colors of tape, so half the class has one color, half has the second color.) Tape the eggs shut.

- Have the children sit in a large circle.
- Pass one egg out to each child.
- Have the children with eggs in color 1 shake together.
- Have the children with eggs in color 2 shake together, etc.
- After each child has experimented with their egg, put on a lively song and have the children shake their egg to the beat of the music.
- They can shake over their heads, behind their backs, roll on the ground, etc.
- When the song is over, discuss what they think is in the eggs. Have them guess.
- Open the eggs and count the candies.
- Have the children sort the candies and make patterns if desired.
- Finally, allow the children to eat the candy!

Questions for the Children:

- What do you think is in the egg?
- What can you do with the egg?
- Which color of egg do you like?
- How many candies are in your egg?
- Can you make a pattern out of the candies?

LESSON EXTENSION IDEAS: Set out a variety of rhythm instruments and have the children choose one to play to the beat of music. Have the children make patterns with rubix cubes or other objects in the classroom.

HOW TO CHECK FOR STUDENT UNDERSTANDING: The teacher will evaluate the students by the way they participate in the lesson. Do they shake the egg to the beat of the music? Are they able to count, sort, and make patterns with the candies?

ACCOMMODATIONS FOR DIVERSE LEARNERS (SPECIAL NEEDS): This lesson will benefit all children. A child with special needs may need help shaking the egg and opening/counting. Seat them close to the teacher.

EVALUATION OF THE LESSON: The teacher will evaluate the lesson by recording the enthusiasm and enjoyment the children displayed during the lesson. If the children have difficulty counting, sorting, and making patterns, this part of the lesson could be eliminated.

ACTIVITY 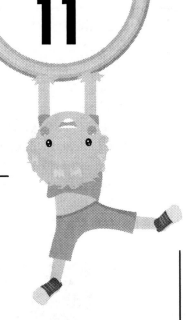 11

SHARK PUPPETS

GOAL:

The children will learn facts about sharks.

OBJECTIVE:

The children will be able to recall information about sharks and make a shark puppet.

Developmental Domain(s) Met:

Physical – The children will use fine motor skills when cutting and assembling the pieces of a shark puppet.

Language and Communication – The children will be able to recall facts about sharks.

Creative – The children will use creativity when making a shark puppet.

Materials Needed:

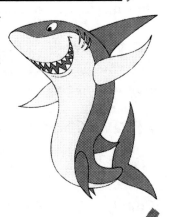

* Book, *Little Shark* by Anne F. Rockwell or any book for young children about sharks
* One legal size white mailing envelope for each child
* One large cut-out shark (poster size)
* Crayons or markers
* Children's scissors
* Glue sticks

Environment (Indoor/Outdoor, Size of Group):

Any size group in the classroom seated at tables.

Procedure:

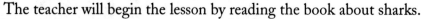

The teacher will begin the lesson by reading the book about sharks.

- Ask the children to recall facts about sharks.
- Write the facts on a large cut out silhouette of a shark.
- Demonstrate how to cut a "V" shape on the end of a white legal size envelope.
- Glue the V-shape to the middle of the envelope as the fin.
- The children will color the shark puppet and add teeth and features.
- The end of the envelope will be cut open, allowing the children to place their hand inside and use as a puppet.

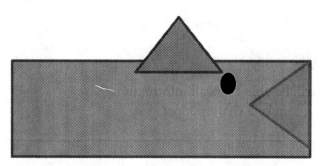

Image courtesy of the author.

Questions for Children:

- Where do sharks live?
- What letter does the word shark begin with?
- What do sharks eat?
- How many kinds of sharks can you name?

LESSON EXTENSION IDEAS: The lesson could be extended by having the children play with their puppets and create a "puppet show" about sharks.

HOW TO CHECK FOR STUDENT UNDERSTANDING: The teacher will write down facts that the children recall about sharks. Each child will be evaluated on their comprehension and ability to recall facts about sharks.

ACCOMMODATIONS FOR DIVERSE LEARNERS (SPECIAL NEEDS): Children with special needs may need help with fine motor skills when cutting and assembling the shark puppet.

EVALUATION OF THE LESSON: The teacher will evaluate the lesson based on the participation of the children and their ability to recall shark facts.

ACTIVITY 12

SINGING BROWN BEAR

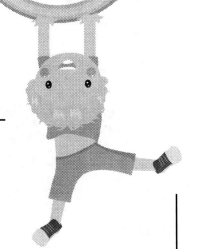

GOAL:
To enjoy music, drama, and literature.

OBJECTIVE:
The children will sing, "Twinkle, Twinkle Little Star" changing the words.

Developmental Domain(s) Met:

Physical – The children will pretend to be animals from the story.
Social/Emotional – The children will take turns and reenact the story.
Language and Communication – The children will sing and communicate with each other.

Materials Needed:

* Book: *Brown Bear, Brown Bear, What Do You See?* by Bill Martin Jr.

Environment (Indoor/Outdoor, Size of Group):

Classroom setting, small group recommended up to 15 children.

Procedure:

The teacher will begin the lesson by reading the book.
- Children will be asked to recall the animals in the story.
- Sing the questions in the story to the tune of "Twinkle, Twinkle Little Star."
- The children will sing the answer to the question referring to which animal is on each page of the book.

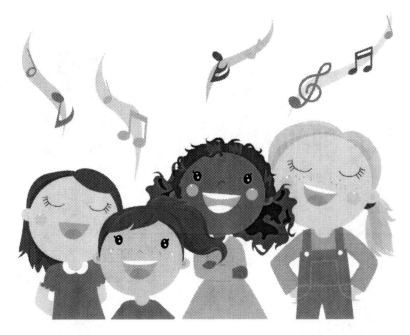

<u>Example:</u>

Teacher sings: Brown bear, brown bear, what do you see?

Children answer by singing: I see a red bird looking at me.

- After the story is read and sung, the children will each choose an animal and sing their part from the story.

Questions for Children:

- What animals were in the story?
- How many animals were in the story?
- Where are these animals' natural habitats?
- What other animals can you name?
- How do you think the skin on the animals feels?

ACCOMMODATIONS FOR DIVERSE LEARNERS (SPECIAL NEEDS): Students with special needs should be seated close to the teacher and have another student help them act out their animal part.

LESSON EXTENSION IDEAS: The children could draw or paint the animal they represented in the story.

HOW TO CHECK FOR STUDENT UNDERSTANDING: The teacher will evaluate the students based on their participation in singing and acting.

EVALUATION OF THE LESSON: The teacher will evaluate the lesson based on the enjoyment the children displayed and if they were able to remember the animals in the story.

Section 5

SUPPLEMENTS

"AM I A BIRD?" – SUPPLEMENT #1

Animals other than birds that can fly.

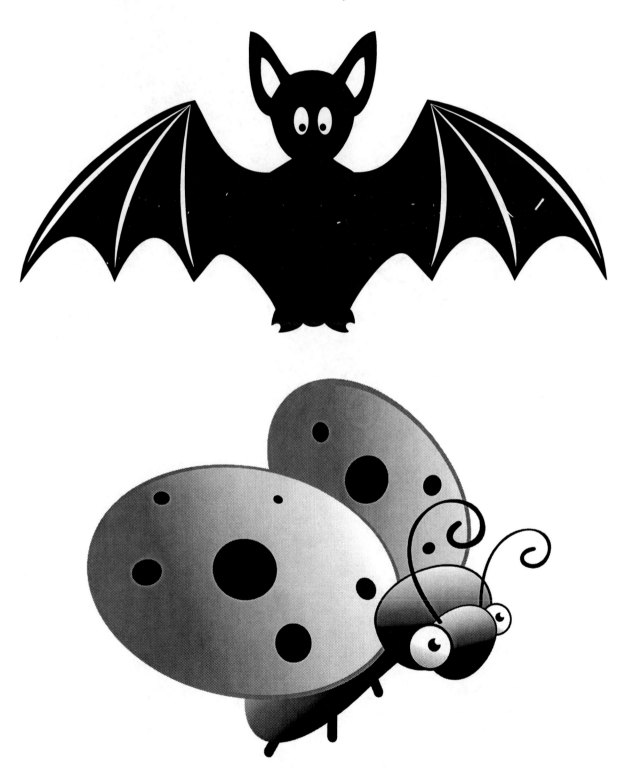

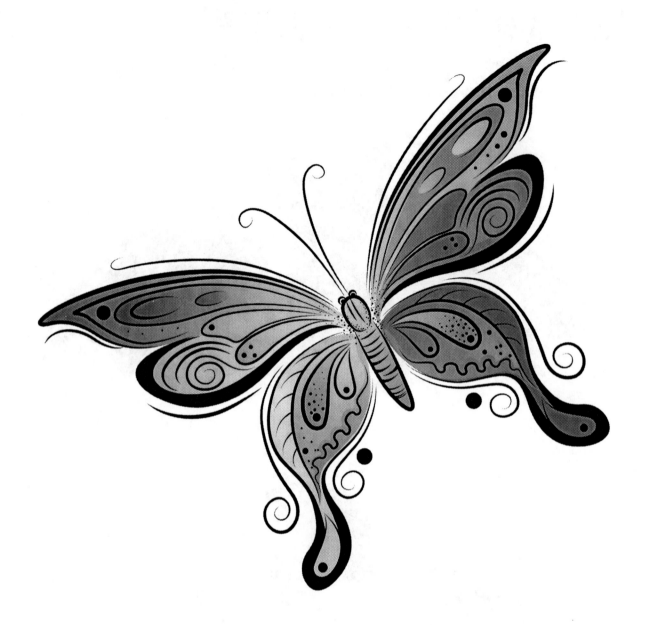

"AM I A FISH?" — SUPPLEMENT #1

Animals other than fish that can swim.

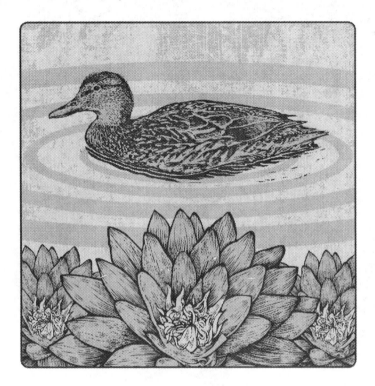

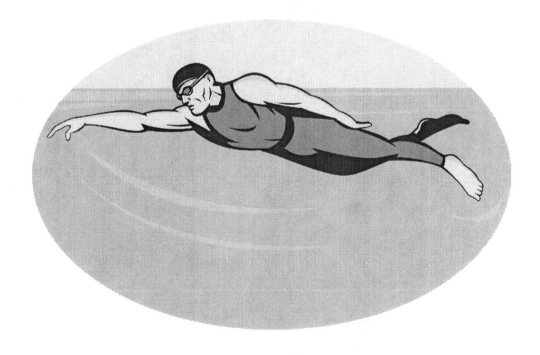

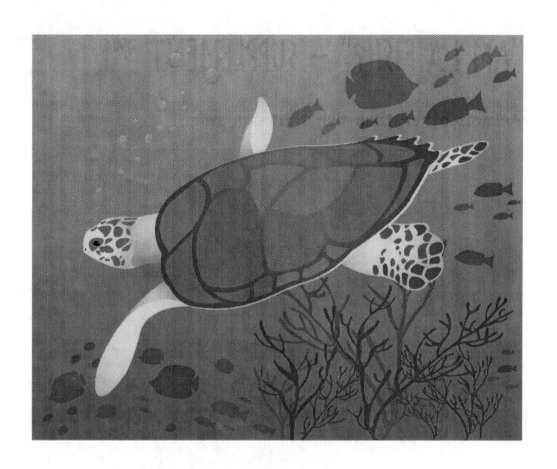

"AM I A MAMMAL?" – SUPPLEMENT #1

Animals that are not mammals.

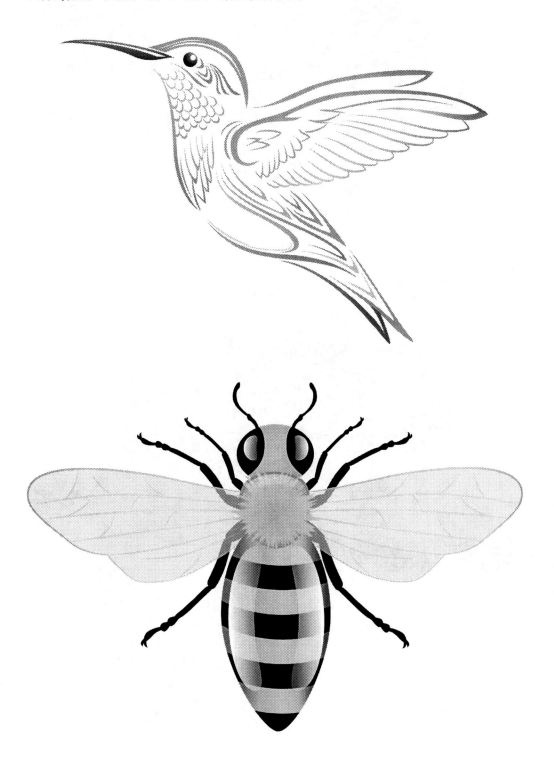

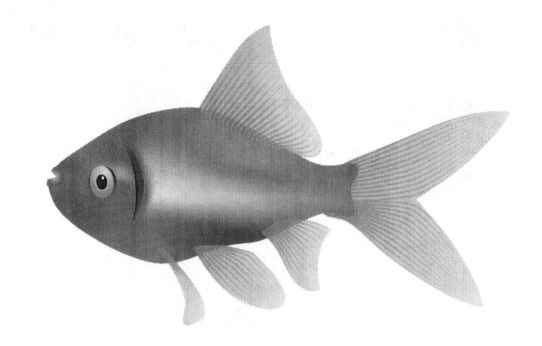

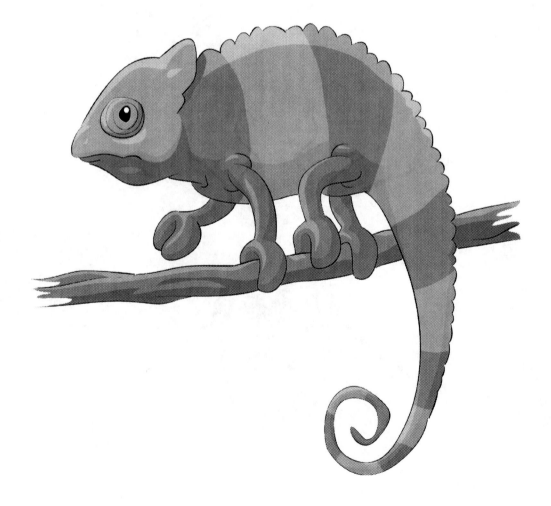

"AM I A PLANT?" — SUPPLEMENT #1

Potted Plants

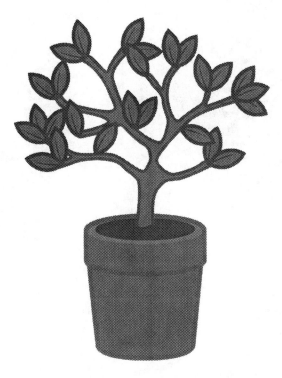

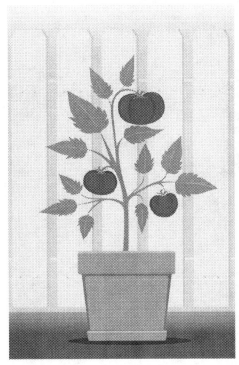

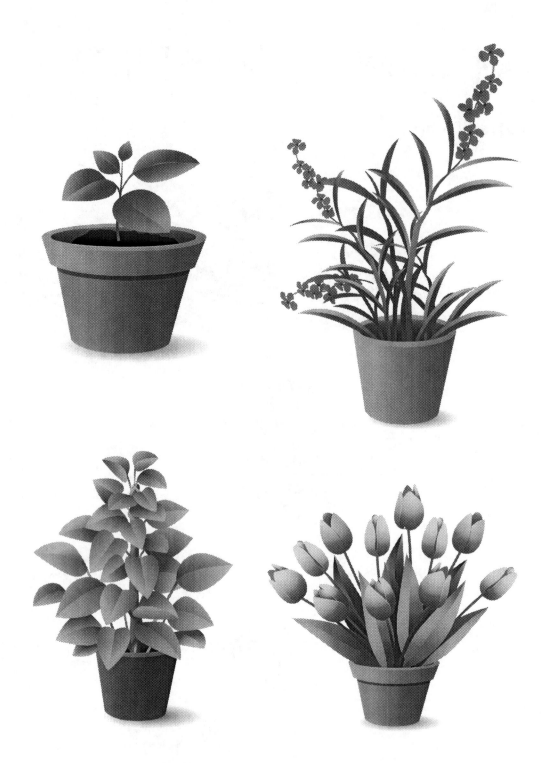

"I HAVE A HEART" — SUPPLEMENT #1

What does a healthy heart need?

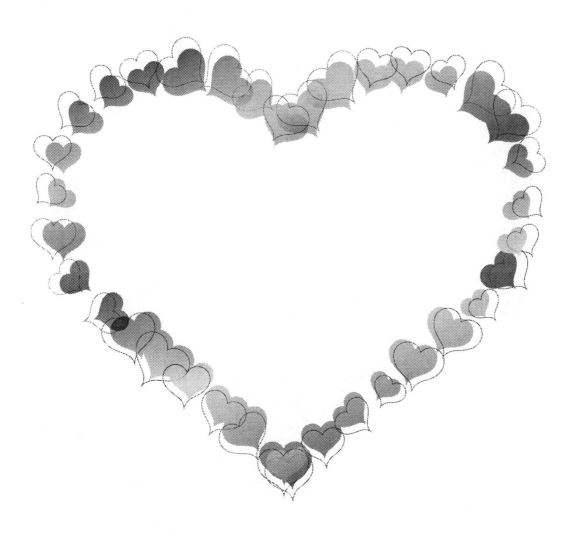

"I TOUCH" – SUPPLEMENT #1

Animal Outlines

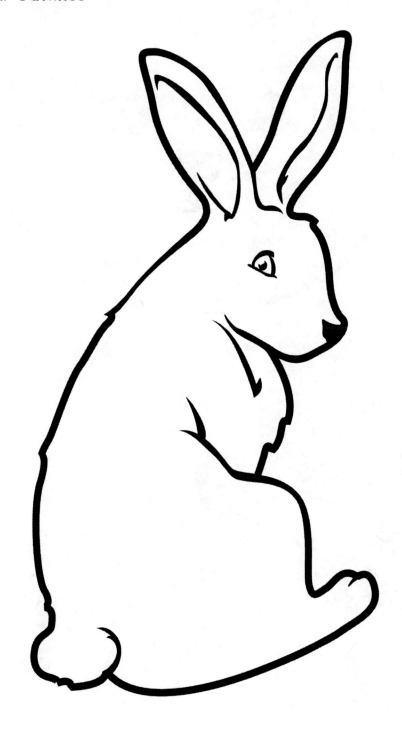

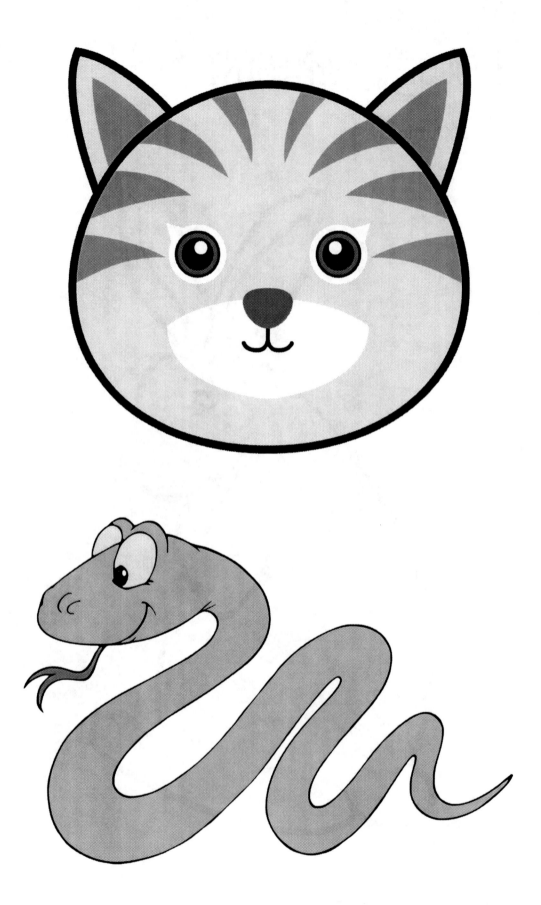

"EVEN OR ODD" – SUPPLEMENT #1

Circle the groups that contain an even number of objects.

1.

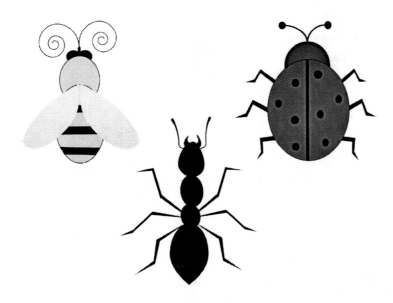

2.

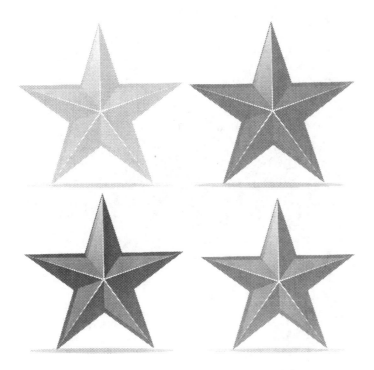

3.

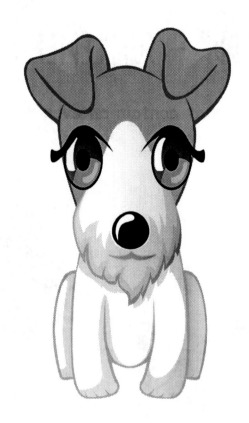

4.

"MORE OR LESS" – SUPPLEMENT #1

Circle the picture that has more animals in it.

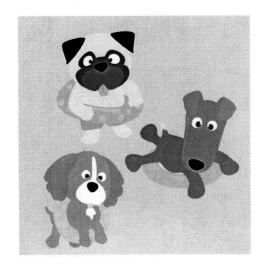 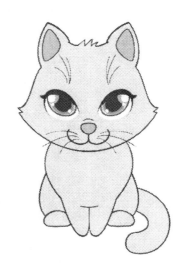

Circle the picture that has less animals in it.

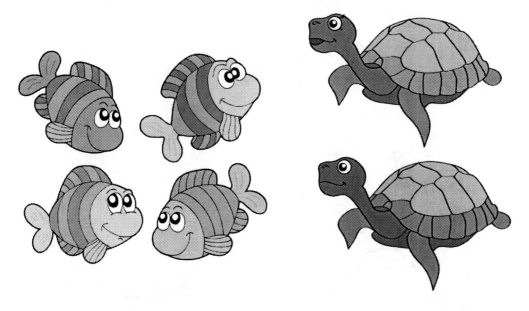

Circle the picture that has more animals in it.

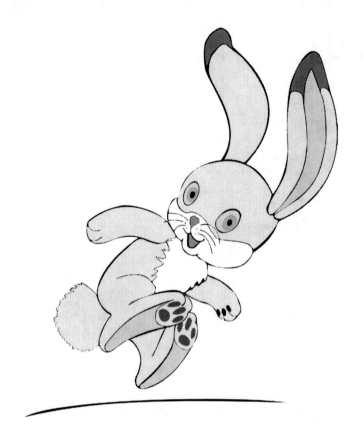

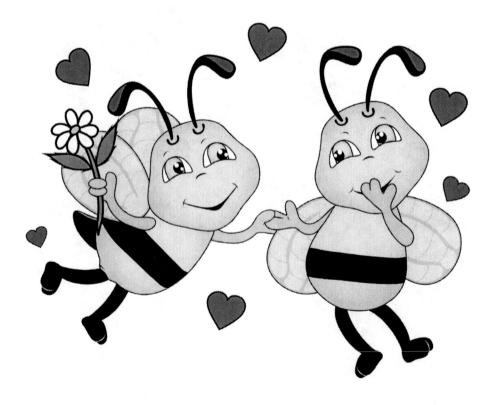

PATTERNS — SUPPLEMENT #1

Continue the pattern on the lines provided.

X O X O X O ___ ___ ___

X O O X O O ___ ___ ___

X X X X ___ ___ ___

O O X X O O X ___ ___ ___

SHAPES — SUPPLEMENT #1

Circle, Triangle, and Square

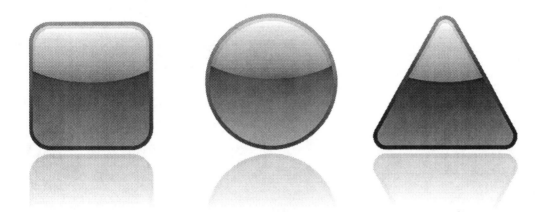

*Under each shape label it Square, Circle, Triangle

"TWO OF A KIND" – SUPPLEMENT #1

Draw a line between the two animals that are the same and make up two of a kind.

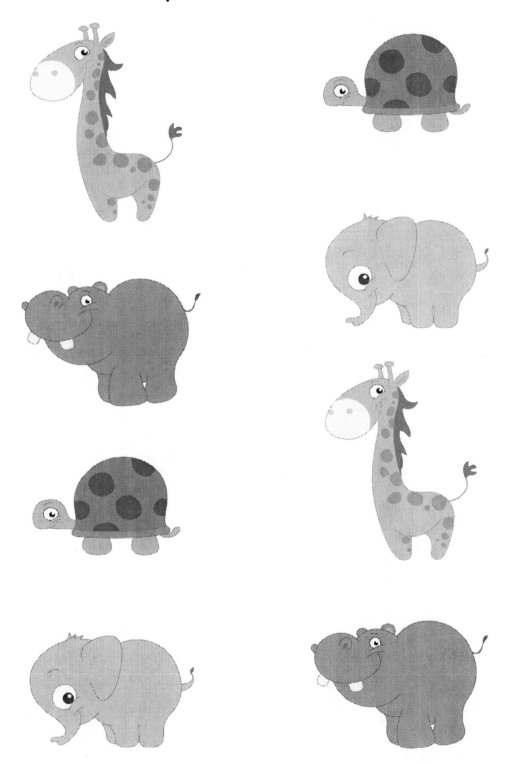